D1274353

CARPAL TUNNEL SYNDROME -- CAUSES, SYMPTOMS, DIAGNOSIS, TREATMENTS AND SURGERY: INDEX OF NEW INFORMATION INCLUDING COMPLICATIONS

AMERICAN HEALTH RESEARCH INSTITUTE

THE WORLD'S BEST RESEARCH BOOKS OF NEW KNOWLEDGE

ABBE PUBLISHERS ASSOCIATION OF WASHINGTON, D.C.
GEORGETOWN 3724 AT 31ST. STREET, N.W.
WASHINGTON, D.C. 20007

ABBE PUBLISHERS: PROFESSIONAL INFORMATION

I.S.B.N. ASSIGNMENTS: 0-941864; 0-88164; 1-55914; 0-7883+

THIS VOLUME: HARDCOVER EDITION: ISBN: 0-7883-11026

THIS VOLUME: PAPERBACK EDITION: ISBN: 0-7883-11034

SPECIAL NOTATION:
WE CONTINUE TO OBEY REQUESTS FOR GENEROUS SPACING ALLOTMENTS TO PERMIT RESEARCH PHYSICIANS, SCIENTISTS, PIONEERS, LABS AND GRADUATE STUDENTS TO INSERT NOTES, DISCOVERIES, NEW DATA AND CURRENT OR NEW REFERENCES TO MAINTAIN THEIR LOGS OF NEW MATERIAL FOR COPYRIGHTS, POSSIBLE PATENTS AND APPLIED TECHNOLOGIES AS WELL AS PROCEDURAL PROTOCOL FOR MASTER'S THESES AND DOCTORAL DISSERTATIONS.

LIBRARY OF CONGRESS CATALOG CARD NUMBER
LIBRARY OF CONGRESS CATALOGING IN PUBLICATION DATA [RC422.C26]

**ARCHIVAL QUALITY REFERENCE BOOK

```ALL ABBE BOOKS AND MONOGRAPHS  may be ordered instantly from Baker & Taylor Books, Blackwell's Book Services, Amazon. Com, Barnes & Noble, Borders Books & Music, The Book House, Academic Book Center, Eastern Book Co, Yankee Book Peddler, Emery-Pratt Co. and many others as listed in Library Reference Sources.

*CORRESPONDENCE ADDRESS: ABBE PUBLISHERS ASSOCIATION
OF WASHINGTON, D.C.: VIRGINIA DIVISION
4111 GALLOWS ROAD
ANNANDALE, VA 22003

**** FAX NUMBER 24 HOURS X 7 DAYS:  (703) 642-5966.
>ACID-FREE EDITIONS <       > SANS ACIDE <        > LIBRE DE ACIDO <

RESEARCH PRODUCES NEW KNOWLEDGE, PROLONGS LIFE,  INCREASES OUR DAILY HAPPINESS, FIGHTS NEW AND OLD DISEASES, LESSENS THE WEARINESS OF LIVING AND ALWAYS SEEKS GREATER PROTECTION AND BETTER HEALTH FOR OUR PRICELESS CHILDREN ---  "THE FLOWERS OF CIVILIZATION" (JCB).
```

TABLE OF CONTENTS

AT THE END:

**YOUR PRIVATE CATALOG OF NEW AND RECENT
BOOKS AND PUBLICATIONS FOR YOUR TOTAL HEALTH,
SURVIVAL, WAR PREVENTION AND WORLD SAVING AS
WELL AS NATIONAL PROGRESS.
      "NEW INFORMATION BEYOND ALL TEXTBOOKS"

GENERAL PREFACE AND SOME PHILOSOPHY

ABBE PUBLISHERS serves science and medicine for mankind in general and specifically for doctors, scientists, medical graduates, biologists, personnel in all technologies and for those aspiring intellects seeking pioneer challenges, new avenues for research and any kind of improvement to put into laboratory, clinical or emergency practice now. The ten leading causes of death in the U.S. create 20 million casualties a year. We have millions more in lame, sickness, disabled in mind and body with the accoutrements of depression, despair and loss of courage and hope. There is unlimited research work for everybody.

Anyone interested in prevention of death, disease, disasters or sickness can easily find important information, new research topics, references, authors and new or rare publications in our published volumes. These monographs as texts serve as REFERENCE BOOKS, RESEARCH INDEXES & RESEARCH GUIDE-BOOKS as well as collected REVIEWS providing the latest of the best research. These professional texts save considerable time and effort in search, study, survey or examination of your special interests or need as well as promotion of knowledge and advancements for mankind.

We specialize in all matters pertaining to HEALTH; WHAT ARE WE WITHOUT GOOD HEALTH. Yet, the world and civilization greatly neglects health care -as proven by the direful absence of health promotion, health maintenance and metabolic balance. Health is still not a world number one priority. How sad. Try to imagine seeking an occupation, love or happiness while in poor health.

These monographs are important to all professions because they represent an UP-TO-DATE INFORMATION SERVICE, NEW RESEARCH COVERAGE AND PROFESSIONAL ANALYSIS of whatever progress is evolving in research. These monographs also serve as a spear for progress into unknown realms.

Librarians, Library Specialists, Library scientists and Information Advisors have these monographs and research books at their disposal whenever they wish to direct doctor or student to special sources for depth and research promise of success. These reference books also give valuable service to all counselors of professions, guidance personnel, professors, research directors, experimental scientists and clinical investigators. Supervisors give these monographs and research indexes to their graduate students to search for THESIS TOPICS. This material adds value and speed to research grant applicants. DISSERTATION topics are easily found in ABBE BOOKs for pioneer research and graduate degrees.

Reference Indexes, Research Monographs, Medical Reviews, Guide-books of Research and Subject Survey Analyses all have their place in the history of field development. These books are a hallmark of the professions and serve as an emblem of progressive research for all mankind.

*EVERYONE MUST HELP IN OUR BATTLES AGAINST SICKNESS AND ALL DISEASES
WHICH ARE QUIETLY WAITING FOR US....

PREFACE TWO - MADE FOR YOU!

Readers not acquainted with fields of science or medicine need not worry or feel intimidated by reading medical or any science articles in any journal. Such literature offers small disadvantage --that of becoming acquainted with the vocabulary therein. This you can do by diligent use of a dictionary to identify the terms used in the articles of your interest or pursuit. Once this is done you have made significant progress.

Learning the limited vocabulary in journal articles gives you a wondrous view of the subject. Hiring a consultant would have been wasteful and expensive. Instead you've done the work by yourself, thus saving time and money and without appointment or disappointment.

Authors of research publications listed herein are important. One often wonders what else this author-scientist-physician may have published, or possess still new but unpublished research. These indexes list all authors so often you will find the same author listed more than once, indicating other publications of this author that may expand your interest or range of intent.

When you find an article you should notice the location of the author and listed address. In times of great need you can write directly to such authors -as in severe illness, near-death scenes or request more new data for a thesis or dissertation degree.

In your literature-subject search, by foot, computer or internet be sure to locate review articles first. Reviews are packed with new data, methods, summaries, controversies and conclusions. They present a sum condensation of years of research in a nutshell for you. You can select and carry research on from there --and becoming a 'new' pioneer!

Intellectually, this civilization is still quite primitive: less than .1% of all people are involved in research -while new diseases as HIV and AIDS creep up on us. Our Indexes help overcome this severe deficit and lead you directly into new discoveries.

HEALTH CARE IS YOUR BEST PRIORITY OF LIFE.

THE GREAT IMPORTANCE OF RESEARCH FOR YOU AND THE WORLD*

1. Nations or citizens without new knowledge, research or arms for health and self-defense become the prey they deserve.
    [Reminder: The law of the Jungle always pertains]

2. Nations without research progress become easy, early victims of disease.

3. Many of us today would not be alive but for antibiotic research.

4. New research prolongs life, health and happiness too.

5. Without new research wars would be always raging somewhere.

6. Research seeks the Holy Grail of heavenly Utopia for mankind.

7. Research is the beating heart of progress for health and longevity.

8. The status of nations is easily determined by their research production.

9. Where there is less research there is more poverty, illness and disease.

10. Research helps babies survive birth & early childhood.

11. Creativity demands constant feeding of new information.

12. Research is the secret gold-mine for civilization.

13. Research is the best offense and defense against any kind of creeping illness, unknown diseases and causes of early deaths.

14. Graduate school research is a wonderful cauldron of and for creativity.

15. The best universities have highly productive research scientists.

16. Research gives great rewards, fame or cheerful life satisfaction.

17. The best students come from highly motivated teachers & scientists.

18. Rapid research promotes publication of Reference Books & Research Indexes: sources of new information beyond current textbooks.

19. Synthesis of new information creates New Knowledge for Progress.

* Excerpts from the book: "Health, Life & Disease Or Why Research Should Be Of Great Importance To All Governments, Consumers, Community leaders, Military Chiefs, Civic and Civilian Leaders, Cosmopolitans and Librarians: A philosophy of life made simple. Dr. John C. Bartone. Abbe Publishers. HC: ISBN 0-7883-1034-6; PB: 1025-4.

11

DEDICATION

TO THE NEW "LABOR VICTIMS"

OF

SCIENCE AND TECHNOLOGY.

PROLOGUE

CARPAL TUNNEL SYNDROME IS A SPECIFIC AILMENT OF THE WRIST. IT SHOULD NOT BE CONFUSED WITH THE DISTRESS SYNDROME CALLED "REPETITIVE STRESS INJURY", OR THE ONE KNOWN AS "CUMULATIVE TRAUMA DISORDER".

'CTS' PRODUCES PAIN AND PARAESTHESIA, REVEALED AS A NUMBING, BURNING OR EVEN A TINGLING SENSATION IN AREAS OF MEDIAN NERVE DISTRIBUTION BECAUSE THE MEDIAN NERVE IS COMPRESSED BY FIBERS AND FILAMENTS OF THE FLEXOR RETINACULUM ABOVE IT.

ONE CAN OFTEN 'DIAGNOSE' SUCH CARPAL TUNNEL PAIN AND DISORDER BY MATCHING AREAS OF THE PAIN WITH THE AREAS OF DISTRIBUTION OF THE MEDIAN NERVE.

REGARDLESS OF ANY PERTINENT DISORDER, PAIN OR THE NAME, THESE CONDITIONS PREVENT NORMAL WORKING AND LIVING. SINCE THESE AFFLICTIONS WORSEN IN TIME, THEY MUST NOT BE TAKEN LIGHTLY OR IGNORED TOO LONG.

THOSE WITH SUCH CONDITIONS AND CONFUSED ABOUT THE ORIGIN AND LOCATION OF SUCH INJURY CAN CONSULT ANY GOOD HUMAN ANATOMY TEXT FOR CONFIRMATION.

ACKNOWLEDGMENTS

We are grateful and indebted to many professional and technical workers and personnel in all parts of the biomedical world. There would be no end to the list of those individuals who should be named as public acknowledgment of their help, guidance, courtesy and even professional rescue at times. We are also appreciative of guidance to leading research physicians and scientists who work without public acclaim and without public gratitude.

These generous and devoted people are certainly a contribution to the world of progress all nations and civilization so desperately need against the constant struggle and battles against poverty, disease and disabling illnesses.

We also wish to thank the many government departments, agencies and federal employees at all levels for their ever so diligent application of time and energy as we strive to help mankind survive with increase of health and happiness.

Many thanks must also be extended to the Directors and Staff of the Library of Medicine for their prodigious productions of the many volumes of biomedical information, services and data resources.

The titles of articles in translation, often used here as well as all over the world, have been performed by the specialists of the Library and to them we happily give full credit.

The Staff of the Library of Congress, the LC Card Catalog and the Cataloging in Publication (CIP) Divisions, full of rare patience of the enduring kind, have been exceeding courteous and professional in their services. They also are a national asset.

INTRODUCTION

A. THE IMPORTANCE OF RESEARCH ON EARTH

A rule of the universe is prevalent, unrelenting deterioration, degradation and decay. This action pertains to everything, organic, inorganic, plant, animal or mineral. All is downward transformation. Therefore we must strive to save, improve, invent, manufacture or create the necessities to maintain what we have, what we are or what we need for health, happiness and longevity. This can be accomplished by research to prevent our sliding backward into early death and oblivion. In brief this process is described by the well-known "PUBLISH OR PERISH" slogan. There is infinitesimal awareness in the general world population of "publish or perish"; yet it is an absolute rule of life that governs us all, knowingly or not.

B. THE IMPORTANCE OF REFERENCES

References are the details of research and help form the stable building blocks of progress for you, your family and all nations.

Survival of self, nations, civilizations and of the world entails many basic ingredients among which the gain, care and use of new knowledge is the principle of intellectual life and progress. The attention, feeding and correct assimilation of new information is gaining increasing 'neglect', concern and dissipation*. There still is no broad, correct spectrum of uniform advance of new data or its application in a continuous, steady and comprehensive manner -as an army marching to its objectives in organized units and goals**. At best, it can be said that bibliographies and reference works lie about as weeds in a dense jungle of loose information including, in these modern times, computerized data.

Librarians are the guiding lights of knowledge to information storage of vast dimension, research guidance and as counselors to student inquires of rare and unknown subjects. Librarians are entrusted with the rare and holy wars of all time: to amass all

matter pertinent to health and our survival and progress from a to z. Life is war and they know it well. Librarians are among the few that understand the necessity, importance and the collection of many sorts and manners of reference material be it in whatever style or diversity for its contents may be eventually in great demand, need or consequence at any time--unexpectedly or otherwise.

Wars have a habit of making old research a national crisis. When World War II began we lost our supply of rubber. Our old chemistry of (neglected) research archives, with new knowledge, permitted synthetic development of substitutes of rubber--and a winning war.

World War II forced us to invent research to produce synthetic quinine which prevented malaria. This rapid research saved many American GIs in the Pacific campaigns (which included some of ABBE's old scientist-authors). Thus, data, old or new, is important.

Reference books, as librarians, also serve as guides in enduring struggles to promote progress for mankind. Reference works, any species thereof, aid, lift and nurture the seeds of human aspiration for creativity for those so able and endowed to seek and explore - and publish --advancements --for country and civilization.

All disciplines, as medical and health, require ultra-new sources of information, especially in presentable form for rapid work, use and assimilation, be it vital or otiose. We have done this for many years.

Scientists are dependent upon librarians to save time, money and energy in literature searches. Our tomes are designed to aid these expectations and prevent engulfment from the tidal waves of world journals presenting and publishing scatter-shot data varieties.

Graduate work of all ages and subjects requires the best books and reference sources. Shortages of reference books and indexes is easily demonstrated: much modern graduate work, theses and dissertations reveal a "re-hash" of known data and information. Symptoms are everywhere; causes are easily diagnosed.

The design, foresight and presentation of ABBE Reference Books and Indexes solves unnecessary need of "rehash". ABBE books offer suggestions for new research for whatever project in demand. These books are marks of world advancements for today and as an emblem of local, national or international progress for tomorrow.

C. PUBLISH OR PERISH !

Nations or individuals that do not create new and publish research indicates a presence of overwhelming problems, as stagnation, a lack of priorities, a miring in the progress of yester-years. Without creativity and publishing new things, deterioration hastens our degeneration. It is not a surprise to us that few people live to a healthy and happy old age! Little, none or slight research means less health care, more child deaths and disease invitations to all.

Life and happiness, with fine health of course, is never, or ever constant --or always good. The seven stages of man reveal man's rainbow of life --with all the infinite problems of neglected health and invading disease. We must teach everyone to learn how to make new contributions to life, society and the world, no matter how small. A mighty mass of new information is constantly needed to make better our life, health, happiness, love, creature comforts and longevity too.

We still have not eliminated wars, diseases, child abuse, drug mis-use, unhappy marriages, sufferings of all types, mental illness, poor health, rampart cancers, universal mal-nutrition, pollution everywhere, poisons and contaminations of food. World populations remain mostly immature. The psyche of man and child is too much neglected. Absence of much needed research progress is anywhere in all peoples and nations. Thus our mission: to produce ultra-new Reference Works, Indexes and Guide-Books. Further, we promote the protection and maintenance of your health and peace of mind.

*Health, Life and Disease --Or Why Research Should Be Of Great Importance to All Governments, Consumers, Community Leaders, Military Chiefs, Civic and Civilian Pioneers, Cosmopolitans and Librarians: A Philosophy of Progress Made Simple. Dr. John C. Bartone. ABBE Publishers Association of Washington, D.C. 3rd Printing. January 2000. Hardcover: ISBN 0-7883-1424-6; Pb: 1023-2.

**Medical Research & The Jungle of Science: A New System For Universal Organization Of All Subjects With Permanent Listing Of All Publications, Authors and Contributions. Dr. John C. Bartone. ABBE Publishers Association of Washington, D.C. 3rd Prtg. January 2000. ISBN 0-7883-1022-4 and 0-7883-1023-2.

INDEX

OF

NEW INFORMATION

AND

PUBLISHED RESEARCH:

AUTHORS,

SUBJECTS,

RESEARCH CATEGORIES

AND

BIBLIOGRAPHICAL REFERENCES

NOTE:

THE NUMBER FOLLOWING
EACH CATEGORY REFERS YOU TO THE
SAME NUMBER LISTED AS A REFERENCE
TITLE IN THE BIBLIOGRAPHY.

CTS = CARPAL TUNNEL SYNDROME
CT   = CARPAL TUNNEL
CTR = CARPAL TUNNEL RELEASE

**100 PATIENTS: CARPAL TUNNEL SYNDROME
013.**

**12 SURGEONS TRAINING: CADAVERA CTR
044.**

**1400 CASES; ENDOSCOPIC DECOMPRESSION
133.**

**1988: U.S. PREVALENCE OF CARPAL TUNNEL S
111.**

**1ST DESCRIPTION; ULNAR ARTERY ANEURYSM
128.**

**2-PORTAL CT RELEASE AND CHANGES
068.**

**2-PORTAL TECHNIQUE: ENDOSCOPIC CTR
046.**

**215 CASES: USE OF MODIFIED CHOW TECHNIQ
049.**

**278 ENDOSCOPIC CTR REVIEW: CHOW TEC
082.**

**3 CASES: CHILDHOOD TYPE OF CTS
061.**

35

40

CTS: TREATMENT FOR
005.

CTS: TROPHIC ULCERS IN
114.

CTS: USE OF STATE WORKERS' COMP DATA
117.

CTS; CLASSICAL CLINICAL SYMPTOMS
022.

CTS; CORRELATION OF SIGNS & TESTS
031.

CTS; MYOFASCIAL MANIPULATIVE RELEASE
069.

CTS; OCCUPATION AND
073.

CTS; OCCUPATION AND
072.

CTS; ROLE OF TRI-D COMPUTERIZED TOMOGR
025.

CTS; SCREENING INDUSTRIAL WORKERS
052.

CTS; SPLINTING FOR
099.

CTS; U.S. SURVEY
111.

45

KASDAN ML ET AL
015.

KATZ JN ET AL
002.

KATZ JN ET AL
087.

KERR CD ET AL
051.

KIROFF GK
072.

KIRSCHBERG GJ ET AL
022.

KONISHIIKE T ET AL
034.

KORRICK SA ET AL
117.

KUNOU M
127.

KUNTZER T
013.

KUZNETSOV NL ET AL
137.

LANG E ET AL
055.

BIBLIOGRAPHIC

REFERENCES

CTS = CARPAL TUNNEL SYNDROME

001
A comparison of endoscopic and open carpal tunnel release.
McDonough JW et al
Wis Med J 1993 Dec; 92(12)675-7.
0 References.

002
A preliminary scoring system for assessing the outcome of carpal tunnel release.
Katz JN et al
J Hand Surg [Am] 1994 Jul; 19(4)531-8.
0 References.

003
A statistical problem in diagnosis of carpal tunnel disease. Letter.
Goodgold J
Muscle Nerve 1994 Dec; 17(12)1490-1.
0 References.

004
A study of the dynamic relationship of the lumbrical muscles and the carpal tunnel.
Yii, NW et al
J Hand Surg [Br] 1994 Aug; 19(4)439-43.
0 References.

005
A treatment for carpal tunnel syndrome: results of follow-up study. Letter.
Bonebrake AR
J Manipulative Physiol Ther 1994 Oct; 17(8) 565-7.
0 References.

006
Acute carpal tunnel syndrome in Hansen's disease.
Gaur SC et al
J Hand Surg [Br] 1994 Jun; 19(3)286-7.
0 References.

007
Acute median neuropathy after wrist trauma. The role of emergent carpal tunnel release.
Mack GR et al
Clin Orthop 1994 Mar; 300:141-6.
0 References.

008
Amyloid polyneuropathy in two German-American families: a new transthyretin variant (Val 107).
Uemichi T et al
J Med Genet 1994 May; 31(5)416-7.
0 References.

009
Bilateral carpal tunnel syndrome in a normal child.
Wilson KM et al
J Hand Surg [Am] 1994 Nov; 19(6)913-4.
0 References.

010
Bilateral compression of the median nerve by supracondylar spurs.
Murali SR et al
J Pediatr Orthop B 1995; 4(1)118-20.
0 References.

011
Carpal tunnel release complicated with acute gout.
Kalia KK et al
Neurosurgery 1993 Dec; 33(6)1102-3.
0 References.

012
Carpal tunnel release using limited direct vision.
Abouzahr MK et al
Plastic Reconstr Surg 1995 Mar; 95(3)534-8.
0 References.

013
Carpal tunnel syndrome in 100 patients: sensitivity, specificity of multi-neurophysiological procedures and estimation of axonal loss of motor, sensory and sympathetic median nerve fibers.
Kuntzer T
J Neurol Sci 1994 Dec 20; 127(2)221-9.
0 References.

014
Carpal tunnel syndrome in mucopolysaccharidoses. A report of four cases in child.
Bona I et al
Electromyogr Clin Neurophysiol 1994 Dec;34(8)471-5.
31 References.

015
Carpal tunnel syndrome not always work related.
Kasdan ML et al
J Ky Med Assoc 1994 Aug; 92(8)295-7.
0 References.

016
Carpal tunnel syndrome surgery may harm
patients' hands. Letter.
Clark GL Jr
Md Med J 1994 Mar; 43(3)237-8.
0 References.

017
Carpal tunnel syndrome with propranolol.
Letter.
Anand KS et al
J Assoc Physicians India 1993 May; 41(5)313.
0 References.

018
Carpal tunnel syndrome, work return
and manipulation therapy. Letter.
Timothy JW
Am Fam Physician 1995 Jan; 51(1)48, 50;
discussion 50, 53, 56-7.
0 References.

019
Carpal tunnel syndrome. A guide to prompt
intervention.
Whitley JM et al
Postgrad Med 1995 Jan; 97(1)89-92; 95-6.
15 References.

020
Carpal tunnel syndrome: a major complication
in hemodialysis patients.
Sivri A et al
Scand J Rheumatol 1994; 23(5)287-90.
0 References.

021
Carpal tunnel syndrome: a frequently
mis-diagnosed common hand problem.
Miller BK
Nurse Pract 1993 Dec; 18(12)52-6.
22 References.

022
Carpal tunnel syndrome: classical clinical
symptoms and electrodiagnostic studies
in poultry workers with hand, wrist and
forearm pain.
Kirschberg GJ et al
South Med J 1994 Mar; 87(3)328-31.
0 References.

023
Carpal tunnel syndrome: evaluation of median
nerve circulation with dynamic contrast-
enhanced MR imaging.
Sugimoto H et al
Radiology 1994 Feb; 190(2)459-66.
0 References.

024
Carpal tunnel syndrome: surgical and non-
surgical treatment. Letter.
Seradge H
J Hand Surg [Am] 1994 Jul; 19(4)704.
0 References

025
Carpal tunnel syndrome: the role of tri-
dimensional computerized tomography.
Cartolari R et al
Chir Organi Mov 1994 Apr-Jun; 79(2)157-62.
0 References.

026
Chiropractic manipulation in carpal tunnel
syndrome.
Valente R et al
J Manipulative Physiol Ther 1994 May; 17
(4)246-9.
0 References.

027
Chronology of separate techniques
for endoscopic carpal tunnel release.
Letter.
Chow J
J Am Osteopath Assoc 1994 Aug; 94(8)628.
0 References.

028
Comparison of multiple frequency vibrometry
testing and sensory nerve conduction measures
in screening for carpal tunnel syndrome in an
industrial setting. Werner RA et al
Am J Phys Med Rehab 1995 Mar-Apr; 74
(2)101-6.
0 References.

029
Comparison of proximal and distal one portal
entry techniques for endoscopic carpal tunnel
release. A cadaver study.
Tsuruta T et al
J Hand Surg [Br] 1994 Oct; 19(5)618-21.
0 References.

030
Conservative management of carpal tunnel
syndrome: a re-examination of steroid injection
and splinting.
Weiss AP et al
J Hand Surg [Am] 1994 May; 19(3)410-5.
0 References.

031
Correlation of clinical sings with nerve
conduction tests in the diagnosis of carpal
tunnel syndrome.
Buch Jaeger N et al
J Hand Surg;[Br] 1995 Dec; 19(6)720-4.
0 References.

032
CTS: carpal tunnel syndrome, the facts
and myths.
Melhorn JM
Kans Med 1994 Sep; 95(9)189-92.
10 References.

033
Cutaneous manifestations of carpal tunnel
syndrome. Letter.
Cox NH et al
J Am Acad Dermatol 1995 Apr; 32(4)682.
0 References.

034
Cystic radio-lucency of carpal bones
in haemodialysis patients. An early indicator
of the onset of carpal tunnel syndrome.
Konishiike T et al
J Hand Surg [Br] 1994 Oct; 19(5)630-5.
0 References.

035
Decision making in detecting abnormal Semmes-
Weinstein monofilament thresholds
in carpal tunnel syndrome.
MacDermid JC et al
J Hand Ther 1994 Jul-Sep; 7(3)1475-6.
0 References.

036
Deficits in the function of small and large
afferent fibers in confirmed cases of CTS.
Letter.
Johnson EW
Muscle Nerve 1995 Jan; 18(1)127-8.
0 References.

037
Detection of modified beta 2-microglobulin
(beta 2m) from amyloid deposits in teno-synovial
tissue of carpal tunnel syndrome
(CTS). Letter.
Odani H et al
Clin Chim Acta 1994 Jun; 227(1-2)209-10.
0 References.

038
Diagnosis and treatment of carpal tunnel
syndrome.
Bartova V et al
Ren Fail 1993; 15(4)533-7.
0 References.

039
Diagnosis and treatment of carpal tunnel
syndrome.   Slater RJ Jr et al
Orthop Rev 1993 Oct; 22(10)1095-105.
72 References.

040
Double incision open technique for carpal tunnel release: an alternative to endoscopic release.
Wilson KM
J Hand Surg [Am] 1994 Nov; 19(6)907-12.
0 References.

041
Dupuytren's disease, carpal tunnel syndrome, trigger finger and diabetes mellitus.
Chammas M et al
J Hand Surg [Am] 1995 Jan; 20(1)109-14.
0 References.

042
Electrical studies as a prognostic factor in the surgical treatment of carpal tunnel syndrome.
Braun RM et al
J Hand Surg [Am] 1994 Nov; 19(6)893-900.
0 References.

043
Electrical studies as a prognostic factor in the surgical treatment of carpal tunnel syndrome.
Braun RM et al
J Hand Surg [Am] 1994 Nov; 19(6)893-900.

044
Endoscopic carpal tunnel release in cadavera. An investigation of the results of 12 surgeons with this training model.
Rowland EB et al
J Bone Joint Surg Am 1994 Feb; 76(2)266-8.
0 References.

045
Endoscopic carpal tunnel release using
the single proximal incision technique.
Agee JM et al
Hand Clin 1994 Nov; 10(4)647-59.
14 References.

046
Endoscopic carpal tunnel release.
Two-portal technique.
Chow JC
Hand Clin 1994 Nov; 10(4)637-46.
13 References.

047
Endoscopic carpal tunnel release.
A current perspective.
Berger RA
Hand Clin 1994 Nov; 10(4)625-36.
48 References.

048
Endoscopic carpal tunnel release.
Bernstein RA
Conn Med 1994 Jul; 58(7)387-94.
30 References.
0 References.

049
Endoscopic carpal tunnel release:
use of the modified Chow technique in 215
cases. Letter.
Rosenfeld JV
Med J Aust 1994 Jun 20; 160(12)799-800.
0 References.

050
Endoscopic median nerve decompression:
early experience.
Skoff HD et al
Plastic Reconstr Surg 1994 Oct; 94(5)691-4.
0 References.

051
Endoscopic versus open carpal tunnel release:
clinical results.
Kerr CD et al
Arthroscopy 1994 Jun; 10(3)266-9.
0 References.

052
Evaluation of current perception threshold
testing as a screening procedure for carpal
tunnel syndrome among industrial workers.
Franzblau A et al
J Occup Med 1994 Sep; 36(9)1015-21.
0 References.

053
Experimental and clinical study of the effect
of naftidrofuryl on the recovery form peripheral
nerve lesions.
Merle M et al
Microsurgery 1994; 15(3)179-86.
0 References.

054
Factors associated with poor outcome following
primary carpal tunnel release in non-diabetic
patients.
Al-Qattan MM et al
J Hand Surg [Br] 1994 Oct; 19(5)622-5.
0 References.

055
Function of thick and thin nerve fibers
in carpal tunnel syndrome before and
after surgical treatment.
Lang E et al
Muscle Nerve 1995 Feb; 18(2)207-15.
0 References.

056
Functional psychomotor deficits associated
with carpal tunnel syndrome.
Jeng OJ et al
Ergonomics 1994 Jun; 37(6)1055-69.
0 References.

057
Giant lipoma of the deep palmar space: mimick-
ing persistent carpal tunnel syndrome.
De Smet L et al Acta Orthop Belg 1994;60(3)334-
5. 058
0 References.

058
Grip strength following carpal tunnel
decompression.
Leach WJ et al
J Hand Surg [Br] 1993 Dec; 18(6)750-2.
0 References.

059
Historical commentary: the wrist flexion test
(Phalen sign).
Vargas Busquets MA
J Hand Surg [Am] 1994 May; 19(3)521.
0 References.

060
How does the neurophysiological assessment
influence the management and outcome of
patients with carpal tunnel syndrome?
Boniface SJ et al
Br J Rheumatol 1994 Dec; 33(12)1169-70.
0 References.

061
Hunter's syndrome as a cause of childhood
type carpal tunnel syndrome: a report of three
cases.
Norman-Taylor F et al
J Pediatr Orthop B 1995; 4(1)106-9.
0 References.

062
Impaired nerve conduction in the carpal tunnel
of platers and truck assemblers exposed to
hand-arm vibration.
Nilsson T et al
Scand J Work Environ Health 1994 Jun;
20(3)189-99.
0 References.

063
Literature review of the usefulness of nerve
conduction studies and electromyography
for the evaluation of patients with carpal
tunnel syndrome. AAEM Quality Assurance
Committee.
Jablecki CK et al
Muscle Nerve 1993 Dec;16(12)1392-414.
165 References.

064
Long-term results of carpal tunnel
decompression.
Assessment of 60 cases.
Haupt WF et al
J Hand Surg [Br] 1993 Aug; 18(4)471-4.
0 References.

065
Lumbrical muscle incursion into the carpal
tunnel during finger flexion.
Cobb TK et al
J Hand Surg [Br]
1994 Aug; 19(4)434-8.
0 References.

066
Magnetic resonance neurography
of the median nerve.
Howe FA et al
Br J Dec; 67(804)1169-72.
0 References.

067
Median nerve injury and the transverse wrist
crease incision in open carpal tunnel release.
Slattery PG
Aust N Z J Surg 1994 Nov; 64(11)768-70.
0 References.

068
Morphologic changes following endoscopic
and two-portal subcutaneous carpal tunnel
release.
Ablove RH et al
J Hand Surg [Am] 1994 Sep; 19(5)821-6.
0 References.

069
Myofascial manipulative release of carpal tunnel syndrome: documentation with magnetic resonance imaging.
Sucher BM
J Am Osteopath Assoc 1993 Dec; 93(12)1273-8.
0 References.

070
Neurophysiological investigation of hands damaged by vibration: comparison with idiopathic carpal tunnel syndrome.
Rosen I et al
Scand J Plast Reconstr Surg Hand Surg
1993 Sep; 27(3)209-16.
0 References.

071
Non-surgically treated carpal tunnel syndrome in the manual worker.
Monsivais JJ et al
Plastic Reconstr Surg 1994 Oct; 94(5)695-8.
0 References.

072
Occupation and the carpal tunnel syndrome.
Letter.
Kiroff GK
Med J Aust 1995 Feb 6; 162(3)166-7.
0 References.

073
Occupation and the carpal tunnel syndrome.
Cullum DE et al
Med J Aust 1994 Nov 7; 161(9)552-4.
40 References.

074
Operative treatment of carpal tunnel syndrome.
Waegeneers S et al
Acta Orthop Belg 1993; 59(4)367-70.
0 References.

075
Outcome following epineurotomy in carpal
tunnel syndrome. a prospective randomized
clinical trial.
Foulkes GD et al
J Hand Surg [Am] 1994 Jul; 19(4)539-47.
0 References.

076
Outcome of carpal tunnel surgery in Washington
State workers' compensation.
Adams ML et al
Am J Ind Med 1994 Apr; 25(4)527-36.
0 References.

077
Outcome of carpal tunnel release in diabetic
patients.
Al-Qattan MM et al
J Hand Surg [Br] 1994 Oct; 19(5)626-9.
0 References.

078
Palpatory diagnosis and manipulative
management of carpal tunnel syndrome.
See comments.
Sucher BM
J Am Osteopath Assoc 1994; 94(8)647-63.
24 References.   Comment in: JAOA 1994
                                Aug; 94(8)632;640

079
Peripheral nerve entrapment caused by motor vehicle crashes.
Coert JH et al
J Trauma 1994 Aug; 37(2)191-4.
0 References.

080
Practice parameter for electro-diagnostic studies in carpal tunnel syndrome: summary statement. American Association of Electrodiagnostic Medicine, American Academy of Neurology, American Academy of Physical Medicine and Rehabilitation.
Muscle Nerve 1993 Dec; 16(12)1390-1.
0 References.

081
Predictive value of nerve conduction measurements at the carpal tunnel.
Nathan PA et al
Muscle Nerve 1993 Dec;16(12)1377-82.
0 References.

082
Prospective review of 278 endoscopic carpal tunnel releases using the modified chow technique.
Nagle D et al
Arthroscopy 1994 Jun; 10(3)259-65.
13 References.

083
Pyridoxine in carpal tunnel syndrome.
Copeland DA et al
Ann Pharmacother 1994 Sep; 28(9)1042-4.
11 References.

084
Quantitative vibrometry and elctro-
physiological assessment in screening
for carpal tunnel syndrome among
industrial workers: a comparison.
Werner RA et al
Arch Phys Med Rehabil 1994 Nov; 75(11)
1228-32.
0 References.

085
Rehabilitation of carpal tunnel surgery patients
using a short surgical incision and an early
program of physical therapy.
Nathan PA et al
J Hand Surg [Am] 1993 Nov; 18(6)1044-50.
0 References.

086
Relation between needle electromyography
and nerve conduction studies in patients
with carpal tunnel syndrome.
Werner RA et al Arch Phys Med Rehabil
1995 Mar; 6(3)246-9.
0 References.

087
Responsiveness of self-reported and objective
measures of disease severity in carpal tunnel
syndrome.
Katz JN et al
Med Care 1994 Nov; 32(11)1127-33.
0 References.

088
**Retracted flexor digitorum profundus tendons:
an uncommon cause of carpal compression
syndrome.**
Vral J et al
Acta Orthop Belg 1994; 60(2)245-7.
0 References.

089
**Reverse Phalen's maneuver as an aid
in diagnosing carpal tunnel syndrome.**
Werner RA et al
Arch Phys Med Rehabil 1994 Jul; 75(7)783-6.
0 References.

090
**Scleromyxoedema associated with synovitis
and myopathy.**
Taylor AL et al
Br J Rheumatol 1994 Sep; 33(9)872-4.
0 References.

091
**Segmental median nerve conduction
measurements discriminate carpal tunnel
syndrome from diabetic polyneuropathy.**
**Hansson S. Muscle Nerve 1995 Apr; 18
(4)445-53.**
0 References.

092
**Sensitivity of the three median-to-ulnar
comparative tests in diagnosis of mild
carpal tunnel syndrome. Letter.**
Preston DC et al
Muscle Nerve 1994 Aug; 17(8)955-6.
0 References.

093
Sensitivity of the various tests for the diagnosis of carpal tunnel syndrome.
Seror P
J Hand Surg [Br] 1994 Dec; 19(6)725-8.
0 References.

094
Sensitivity of various electrophysiologic studies for the diagnosis of carpal tunnel syndrome.
Letter.
Seror P
Muscle Nerve 1993 Dec;16(12)1418-9.
0 References.

095
Sensory disturbances after two-portal endoscopic carpal tunnel release: a preliminary report.
Arner M et al
J Hand Surg [Am] 1994 Jul; 19(4)548-51.
0 References.

096
Sensory neural conduction of median nerve from digits and palm stimulation in carpal tunnel syndrome.
Rossi S et al
Electroencephalogr Clin Neurophysiol 1994 Oct; 93(5)330-4.
0 References.

097
Serum hyaluronic acid and interleukin-6 as possible markers of carpal tunnel syndrome in chronic hemodialysis patients.
Takasu S et al
Artif Organs 1994 Jun; 18(6)420-4.
0 References.

098
Significance of incomplete release of the distal portion of the flexor retinaculum. Implications for endoscopic carpal tunnel surgery.
Cobb TK et al
J Hand Surg [Br] 1994 Jun; 19(3)283-5.
0 References.

099
Splinting for carpal tunnel syndrome: in search of the optimal angle.
Burke DT et al
Arch Phys Med Rehabil 1994 Nov; 75(11)1241-4.
0 References.

100
Subjective and employment outcome following secondary carpal tunnel surgery.
Strasberg SR et al
Ann Plast Surg 1994 May; 32(5)485-9.
0 References.

101
Successful treatment response of granuloma annulare and carpal tunnel syndrome to chlorambucil.
Winkelmann RK et al
Mayo Clin Proc 1994 Dec; 69(12)1163-5.
0 References.

102
Surgical management of recurrent carpal tunnel syndrome.
Chang B et al
J Hand Surg [Br] 1993 Aug; 18(4)467-70.
0 References.

103
Surgical treatment of carpal tunnel syndrome in patients exposed to vibration from handheld tools.
Bostrom L et al
Scand J Plast Reconstr Surg Hand Surg
1994 Jun; 28(2)147-9.
0 References.

104
Temperature effects on nerve conduction studies in patients with carpal tunnel syndrome.
Baysal Al et al
Acta Neurol Scand 1993 Sep; 88(3)213-6.
0 References.

105
The carpal tunnel syndrome. Relationship between median distal motor latency and graded results of needle electromyography.
Murga L et al
Electromyogr Clin Neurophysiol 1994
Sep;34(6)377-83.
0 References.

106
The carpal-compression test. An instrumented device for diagnosing carpal tunnel syndrome.
Durkan JA Orthop Rev 1994 Jun; 23(6)522-5.
0 References.

107

The influence of age on distal latency comparison in carpal tunnel syndrome.
Hennessey WJ et al
Muscle Nerve 1994 Oct; 17(10)1215-7.
0 References.

108

The median-ulnar latency difference studies are comparable in mild carpal tunnel syndrome.
Preston DC et al
Muscle Nerve 1994 Dec; 17(12)1469-71.
0 References.

109

The relationship between body mass index and the diagnosis of carpal tunnel syndrome. Letter.
Nathan PA et al
Muscle Nerve 1994 Dec; 17(12)1491-3.
0 References.

110

The role of imaging in the diagnosis of carpal tunnel syndrome.
Rosenbaum RB
Invest Radiol 1993 Nov; 28(11)1059-62.
0 References.

111

The U.S. prevalence of self-reported carpal tunnel syndrome: 1988 National Health Interview Survey Data.
Tanaka S et al
Am J Public Health 1994 Nov; 84(11)1846-8.
0 References.

112
The value of magnetic resonance imaging in carpal tunnel syndrome.
Seyfert S et al
J Neurol 1994 Dec; 242(1)41-6.
0 References.

113
Transection of the motor branch of the ulnar nerve as a complication of two-portal endoscopic carpal tunnel release: a case report.
De Smet L et al
J Hand Surg [Am] 1995 Jan; 20(1)18-9.
0 References.

114
Trophic ulcers in the carpal tunnel syndrome.
Arajuo AQ et al
Arq Neuropsiquiatr 1993 Sep; 51(3)386-8.
0 References.

115
Type 4 median nerve entrapment after elbow dislocation.
Al-Qattan MM et al
J Hand Surg [Br] 1994 Oct; 19(5)613-5.
0 References.

116
Unilateral carpal tunnel syndrome and space-occupying lesions.
Nakamichi, K et al
J Hand Surg [Br] 1993 Dec; 18(6)748-9.
0 References.

117
use of state workers' compensation data
for occupational carpal tunnel syndrome
surveillance: a feasibility study in
Massachusetts.
Korrick SA et al
Am J Ind Med 1994 Jun; 25(6)837-50.
0 References.

118
Using pyridoxine to treat carpal tunnel
syndrome.
Randomized control trial.
Spooner GR et al
Can Fam Physician 1993 Oct; 39:2122-7.
0 References.

119
Validation of occupational hand use categories.
Nathan PA et al
J Occup Med 1993 Oct; 35(10)1034-42.
0 References.

120
Vibration sensibility testing in the workplace.
Day-to-day reliability.
Rosecrance JC et al
J Occup Med 1994 Sep; 36(9)1032-7.
0 References.

121
Vibrometry testing for carpal tunnel syndrome:
a longitudinal study of daily variations.
White KM et al
Arch Phys Med Rehabil 1994 Jan; 75(1)25-8.
0 References.

122
Weight of evidence links obesity, fitness
to carpal tunnel syndrome. Companies
implementing wellness programs experience
a reduction in CTS incidence.
Allen CW Jr
Occup Health Saf 1993 Nov; 62(11)51-2.
0 References.

123
Why do some people develop two or more
inflammatory conditions (ie, carpal tunnel
syndrome, Dupuytren's contracture, trigger
finger, etc) without any clear-cut etiologic
factor(s) being present?
J Occup Med 1994 Mar; 36(3)295-6.
0 References.

124
Wisconsin occupational carpal tunnel syndrome
surveillance; the incidence of surgically treated
cases.
Hanrahan LP et al
Wis Med J 1993 Dec; 92(12)685-9.
0 References.

125
[Ambulatory surgical therapy of carpal tunnel
syndrome. Letter]
Hoffmann R
Chirurg 1994 Oct; 65(10)Suppl 221;
discussion 222. In German.
0 References.

126
[Ambulatory surgical therapy of carpal tunnel syndrome. Letter]
Bruser P
Chirurg 1994 Oct; 65(10) Suppl 221-2; discussion 222. In German.
0 References.

127
[An anatomic study of the carpal tunnel syndrome for endoscopic carpal tunnel release]
Kunou M
Nippon Seikeigeka Gakkai Zasshi 1994 Oct; 68(10)878-84. In Jpn with English abstract.
0 References.

128
[Aneurysm of the ulnar artery as etiology of carpal tunnel syndrome: case report and first description]
Fricker R et al
Handchir Mikrochir Plast Chir 1994 Sep; 26(5)268-9. In German with English abstract.
0 References.

129
[Carpal tunnel syndrome. Can it still be a controversial topic?]
Foucher G et al
Chirurgie 1993-94; 119(1-2)80-4. In French with English abstract.
0 References.

130
[Chronic polyarthritis and carpal tunnel syndrome. Results of follow-up]
Sturm T et al
Z Rheumatol 1995 Jan-Feb; 54(1)56-62.
In German with English abstract.
0 References.

131
[Clinical aspects and therapy of carpal tunnel syndrome]
Piotrowski WP et al
Z Orthop Ihre Grenzgeb 1994 Sep-Oct; 132(5)432-6. In German with English abstract.
0 References.

132
[Complications after endoscopic carpal tunnel decompression]
Herren DB et al
Z Unfallchir Versicherungsmed 1994 Jul; 87(2)120-7.
In German with English abstract.

133
[Endoscopic decompression of the median nerve in the carpal tunnel. Apropos of 1400 cases]
Friol JP et al
Ann Chir Main Memb Super 1994; 13(3)162-71.
In French with English abstract.
0 References.

134
[Sensory potential of the ring finger. Its value in the electromyographic diagnosis of carpal tunnel syndrome. Letter]
Metral S
Ann Chir Main Memb Super 1994; 13(5)354-7.
0 References.

135
[The efficacy of naftidrofuryl on unexpected autonomic symptoms following carpal tunnel surgery]
Chaise F et al
Ann Chir Main Memb Super 1994; 13(3)214-21.
In French with English abstract.
0 References.

136
[The future of the carpal tunnel syndrome]
Saraux A et al
Rev Rhum Ed Fr 1994 Jan; 61(1)3-8. In French.
32 References.

137
[The pathogenesis of tunnel syndromes]
Kuznetsov NL et al
Zh Nevropatol Psikhiatr Im S S Korsakova
1993; 93(4)34-6.
In Russian with English abstract.
0 References.

138
[Validity of clinical signs and provocative tests in carpal tunnel syndrome]   Buch N et al
Rev Chir Orthop Reparatrice Appar Mot 1995;
80(1)14-21. In French with English abstract.
0 References.

139
[With respect to Tinel and Phalen's signs]
Martinez-Albaladejo M et al
An Med Interna 1994 Jan; 12(1)21-4.
In Spanish with English abstract.
0 References.

EPILOGUE AND FARE--THEE--WELL!

SCIENCE AND TECHNOLOGY SOMETIMES

CREATE MORE THAN HUMAN BENEFITS.

WE NEED TIME TO CORRECT NATIONAL

ERRORS THAT COME WITH THE BENEFITS!

RESEARCH AND PROGRESS FOR ALL MANKIND

NEW REFERENCE BOOKS & RESEARCH INDEXES
2001 TO 2002 (to be continued)

OUR CONCERN IS YOUR HEALTH, AND THAT OF THE WORLD !
GOOD HEALTH IS OUR GREATEST WEALTH !
WHAT ARE WE, PERSON, BABY, CHILD OR COUNTRY
---WITHOUT GOOD HEALTH?
OUR INDEXES PROMOTE HEALTH, PEACE AND HAPPINESS.

*

FAX ORDERS TO (703) 642-5966 : OPEN 24 HOURS A DAY, 7 DAYS A WEEK

*

OR WRITE TO: ABBE PUBLISHERS ASSOCIATION OF WASHINGTON, D.C.

4111 GALLOWS ROAD : VIRGINIA DIVISION
ANNANDALE, VIRGINIA USA 22003

BIOTERRORISM and Biology of Botulism (Clostridium Botulinum): Index of New Information and Guide-Book for Consumers, Reference and Research. December 2001. Cloth, 57.50: ISBN 0-7883-2710-0; PB is 50.50: ISBN 0-7883-2711-9. 175p. Dr. John C. Bartone.
(See also title of Terrorism).

TERRORISM & Health Science Affairs: Index of New Information and Guide-Book for Consumers, Reference and Research. November 2001. Cloth, 57.50: ISBN 0-7883-2548-5; PB is 50.50: ISBN 0-7883-2549-3. 175p. Dr. John C. Bartone. (See also titles of Bioterrorism).

BIOTERRORISM OF SMALLPOX (Variola Virus): Index of New Information and Guide-Book for Consumers, Reference and Research. Nov 2001. Cloth, 57.50: ISBN 0-7883-2588-4; PB is 50.50: ISBN 0-7883-2589-2. 175p. Dr. John C. Bartone. (See also title of Terrorism).

BIOTERRORISM OF PLAGUE (Yersinia Infections): Index of New Information and Guide-Book for Consumers, Reference and Research. November 2001. Cloth, 57.50: ISBN 0-7883-2630-9; PB is 50.50: ISBN 0-7883-2631-7. 175p. Dr. John C. Bartone. (See also title of Terrorism).

BIOTERRORISM OF ANTHRAX (Bacillus anthracis): Index of New Information and Guide-Book for Consumers, Reference and Research. November 2001. Cloth, 57.50: ISBN 0-7883-2564-7; PB is 50.50: ISBN 0-7883-2565-5. 175p. Dr. John C. Bartone. (See also title of Terrorism).

BIOTERRORISM, THREATS AND BIOLOGY OF TOXINS: Index of New Information and Guide-Book for Consumers, Reference and Research. December 2001. Cloth 57.50: ISBN 0-7883-2698-8; PB is 50.50: ISBN 0-7883-2699-6. 175p. Dr. J. C. Bartone (See also title of Terrorism).

WAR --Analysis, Research, Policy and Politics with Progress: Index of New Information for Reference, Research and Archives. April 2002. Cloth 67.50: ISBN 0-7883-2430-6; PB is 57.50: ISBN 0-7883-2431-4. 175p. Science & Life Consultants.

Coenzyme Q - Ubiquinone: Index of New Information and Guide-Book for Consumers, Reference and Research. March 2002. Cloth 57.50: ISBN 0-7883-2498-5; PB is 47.50: 0-7883-2499-3; 175p. Dr. Adolph A. Smithson.

Vitamin G - Riboflavin: Index of New Information and Guide-Book for Consumers, Reference and Research. March 2002. Cloth, 57.50; ISBN 0-7883-2486-1; PB is 47.50: ISBN 0-7883-2487-X. 175p. Dr. Adolph A. Smithson.

Vitamin H - Biotin: Index of New Information and Guide-Book for Consumers, Reference and Research. April 2002. Cloth, 57.50: ISBN 0-7883-2504-3; PB is 47.50: ISBN 0-7883-2505-1. 175p. Dr. Adolph A. Smithson.

Vitamin M - Folic Acid: Index of New Information and Guide-Book for Consumers, Reference and Research. June 2002. Cloth, 57.50: ISBN 0-7883-2506-X; PB is 47.50: ISBN 0-7883-2507-8. 175p. Dr. Adolph A. Smithson.

Vitamin PP - Niacinamide: Index of New Information and Guide-Book for Consumers, Reference and Research. May 2002. Cloth, 57.50:ISBN 0-7883-2508-6; PB is 47.50: ISBN 0-7883-2509-4. 175p. Dr. Adolph A. Smithson.

Vitamin P Complex - Bioflavonoids: Index of New Information and Guide-Book for Consumers, Reference and Research. May 2002. Cloth, 57.50: 0-83-2524-8; PB is 47.50: ISBN 0-7883-2525-6. 175p. Dr. Adolph A. Smithson.

Vitamin B-T: Carnitine: Index of New Information and Guide-Book for Consumers, Reference and Research. June 2002. Cloth, 57.50:ISBN 0-7883-2526-4; PB is 47.50: ISBN 0-7883-2527-2. 175p. Dr. Adolph A Smithson.

FAX ORDERS TO: (703) 642-5966: OPEN 24 HOURS A DAY X 7 DAYS A WEEK

RESEARCH AND PROGRESS FOR ALL MANKIND

NEW REFERNCE BOOKS AND RESEARCH INDEXES

PLANET EARTH IGNORES THE IMPORTANCE OF RESEARCH

Choking and Air-Way Obstructions: Index of New Information for Consumers, Reference and Research. May 202. Cloth, 57.50: ISBN 0-7883-2546-9; PB is 47.50: ISBN 0-7883-2547-7. 175p. Dr. Joanne C. Silvester.

Food Alterations & Contaminations: Index of New Information and Guide-Book for Consumers, Reference and Research. April 2002. Cloth, 57.50: ISBN 0-7883-2550-7; PB is 47.50: ISBN 0-7883-2551-5. 175p. Dr. Theodore K. Sloan.

Health Dangers of Free Radical Chemistry: Index of New Information and Guide-book for Consumers, Reference and Research. April 2002. Cloth, 57.50: ISBN 0-7883-2552-3; PB is 47.50: ISBN 0-7883-2553-1. 175p. Dr. Alfred H Towson.

Elbow - Its injuries and Cubital Tunnel Syndrome: Index of New Information and Guide-Book for Consumers, Reference and Research. May 2002. Cloth, 57.50: ISBN 0-7883-2554-X; PB is 47.50: ISBN 0-7883-2555-8. 175p. Dr. Doris Nash Tabor.

Neuro-Protective Agents & Therapeutic Uses: Index of New Information and Guide-Book for Consumers, Reference and Research. May 202. Cloth, 57.50: ISBN 0-7883-2566-3; PB is 47.50: ISBN 0-7883- 2567-1. 175p. Dr. Carole E. Spandola.

LASIK Eye Surgery (Laser in Situ) (Kerato-mileusis): Index of New Information and Guide-Book for Consumers, Reference and Research. February 2002. Cloth, 57.50: ISBN 0-7883-2500-0; PB is 47.50: ISBN 0-2501-9. 175p. Dr. Harvey K. Melbone.

Mis-Conduct and Illegal Behavior in Science & Medicine: Index of New Information and Guide-Book For Consumers, Reference and Research. May 2002. Cloth, 57.50: ISBN 0-7883-2568-X; PB is 47.50: ISBN 0-7883-2569-8. 175p. Dr.Carmella T. Dellabella.

Science on Planet Earth -Progress, Comments, Controversy, Editorials and Economics: Index of New Information and Guide-Book for Consumers, Reference and Research. May 2002. Cloth, 57.50: ISBN 0-7883-2406-3; PB is 47.50: ISBN 0-7883-2407-1. 175p. Dr. Carmella T. Dellabella.

FAX ORDERS TO: (703) 642-5966: OPEN 24 HOURS A DAY X 7 DAYS A WEEK

BIBLIOGRAPHIC INFORMATION FOR ALL NATIONS

4

RESEARCH AND PROGRESS FOR ALL MANKIND

NEW REFERENCE BOOKS AND RESEARCH INDEXES

RICH NATIONS... PERFORM MORE RESEARCH...
...THAN POOR NATIONS

Microbiology of Air: Index of New Information and Guide-book for Consumers, Reference and Research. March 2002. Cloth, 57.50: ISBN 0-7883-2296-6; PB is 47.50: ISBN 0-7883-2297-4. 175p. Dr. Michael I. Mayer.

Movement Discomfort & Disorders (Dyskinesias): Index of New Information for Consumers, Reference and Research. June 2002. Cloth, 57.50: ISBN 0-7883-2408-X; PB is 47.50: ISBN 0-7883-2409-8. 175p. Dr. Jonathan L. Blakiston.

Cancer and Chromosome Aberrations: Index of New Information for Consumers, Reference and Research. June 2002. Cloth, 57.50: ISBN 0-7883-2420-9; PB is 47.50: ISBN 0-7883-2421-7. 175p. Dr. John C. Bartone.

Vegetarianism For Family Health & Longevity: Index of New Information for Consumers, Reference and Research. January 2002. Cloth, 57.50: ISBN 0-7883-2422-5; PB is 47.50: ISBN 0-7883-2423-3. 175p. Dr. Victoria Marie McQueen.

Life Stress, Distress and Depression in the psychological garden of mental illness and the complex variations in human activities: Index of New Information for Consumers, Reference and Research. May 2002. Cloth, 57.50: ISBN 0-7883-2424-1; PB is 47.50: ISBN 0-7883-2425-X. 175p. Dr. Chester O. Donovan.

Appetite Disturbances & Disorders - Early behavior and hyperphagia. Index of New Information for Consumers, Reference and Research. May 2002. Cloth, 57.50: ISBN 0-7883-2426-8; PB is 47.50: ISBN 0-7883-2427-6. 175p. Marilyn Osborne Agresti.

Obesity & Anti-obesity Agents: Index of New Information for Consumers, Reference and Research. March 2002. Cloth, 57.50: ISBN 0-7883-2432-2; PB is 47.50: ISBN 0-7883-2433-0. 175p. Dr. Joseph R. Richie.

HIV Epidemic Continues in the United States: Index of New Information for Consumers, Reference and Research. January 2002. Cloth, 57.50: ISBN 0-7883-2442-X; PB is 47.50: ISBN 0-7883-2443-8. 175p. Dr. Silvester V. Polanta.

FAX ORDERS TO: (703) 642-5966: OPEN 24 HOURS A DAY X 7 DAYS A WEEK

BIBLIOGRAPHIC INFORMATION FOR ALL NATIONS

RESEARCH AND PROGRESS FOR ALL MANKIND

NEW REFERENCE BOOKS AND RESEARCH INDEXES

RESEARCH: THE MOST NEGLECTED AREA IN THE ENTIRE WORLD

AIDS & HIV Long term survivors --Analysis and Results: Index of New Information and Guide-Book for Consumers, Reference and Research. January 2002. Cloth, 57.50: ISBN 0-7883-2444-6; PB is ISBN 0-7883- 2445-4. 175p. Dr. Silvester V. Polanta.

Human Anatomy with Over-Use Syndromes and Cumulative Trauma Disorders: Index of New Information and Guide-Book for Consumers, Reference and Research. February 2002. Cloth 57.50: ISBN 0-7883-2446-2; PB is 47.50: ISBN 0-7883-2447-0. 175p. Dr. Jean Gray Yodell.

Biogenesis of Life- In fact, theory and controversy: Index of New Information and Guide-Book for Consumers, Reference and Research. April 2002. Cloth, 57.50: ISBN 0- 7883- 2458-6; PB is 47.50: ISBN 0-7883-2459-4. 175p. Dr. Hans Hermann Schmidt.

Evolution & The Origin of Life: Index of New Information and Guide-Book for Consumers, Reference and Research. April 2002. Cloth, 57.50: ISBN 0-7883-2476-4; PB is 47.50: ISBN 0-7883-2477-2. 175p. Hans Hermann Schmidt.

Over-weight, Over-eating, obesity and morbidity in America: Index of New Information and Guide-Book for Consumers, Reference and Research. April 2002. Cloth, 57.50: ISBN 0-7883-2490-X; PB is 47.50: ISBN 0-7883- 2491-8. 175p. Dr. Tyrone T. Powers.

Sleep -Deficiency, Deprivations, Disturbances and Disorders: Index of New Information and Guide-Book for Consumers, Reference and Research. February 2002. Cloth, 57.50: ISBN 0-7883-2494-2; PB is 47.50: ISBN 0-7883- 2495-0. 175p. Dr. Jamin K. Mottolova.

African-Americans -Analysis, Behavior, Progress and Results: Index of New Information and Guide-Book for Consumers, Reference and Research. February 2002. Cloth 57.50: ISBN 0-7883-1484-X; PB is 47.50: ISBN 0-7883- 1495-5. 175p. Dr. Jeannette O. Wilson.

Humor, Mirth & Mischief at Life and Philosophy: Snappy lines for Home, Office and parties or for everyday laughs. Cloth, 34.95: ISBN 0-7883-1058-5; PB is 24.95: ISBN 0-7883-1059-3. 150p. Dr. Vito Vanderbilt.

FAX ORDERS TO: (703) 642-5966: OPEN 24 HOURS A DAY X 7 DAYS A WEEK

BIBLIOGRAPHIC INFORMATION FOR ALL NATIONS

RESEARCH AND PROGRESS FOR ALL MANKIND

NEW REFERENCE BOOKS AND RESEARCH INDXES

RESEARCH IS OUR BEST SALVATION AGAINST DISEASE & FILTH

Anger and Rage --Analysis and Conclusions of Life of Modern Times: Index of New Information and Guide-Book for Consumers, Reference & Research. February 2002. Cloth, 57.50: ISBN 0-7883-2342-3 PB is 47.50: ISBN 0-7883-2343-1. Am Health Research.180p.

Cancer Epidemics Are World-Wide and Affecting All Parts of the Human Body: Index of New Information and Guide-Book for Consumers, Reference and Research. March 2002. Cloth, 67.50: ISBN 0-7883-2404-7; PB is 57.50: ISBN 0-7883-2405-5. 175p. Dr. John C. Bartone.

Coffee –America's Favorite All-Day Beverage and Relaxation Drink: Index of New Information and Guide-Book for Consumers, Reference and Research. May 2002. Cloth 57.57: ISBN 0-7883-2594-9; Pb is 47.50: ISBN 0-7883-2595-7. 180P. Dr. Judy G. Hanson.

American Attitudes: U.S. Register A to Z: Index and Analysis of New Information and Guide-Book for Consumers, Reference and Research. 5 Volumes: Cloth is $ 425.00; ISBN for 5 volumes is 0-7883-2876-X; Pb of 5 volumes is $ 375.00; ISBN 0-7883-2877-8. *Each volume: Cloth is $ 85.00 each; Pb is $ 75.00 each.

BIOTERRORISM–A Biological and Medical Bibliography of 1200 Citations for Reference, Research and Preparedness. June 2002. Cloth is $ 85.50, ISBN 0-7883-2707-0; PB is $ 75.50, ISBN 0-7883-2708-9. Dr. John C. Bartone, 275p.

FETAL ALCOHOL SYNDROME –THE MAN-MADE DISEASE FOR BABIES AND CHILDREN: INDEX OF NEW INFORMATION. 3rd Edition. September 2002. Cloth is $ 57.50, ISBN 0-7883-2734-8; Pb is 47.50, ISBN 0-7883-2735-6. Dr. John C. Bartone. 160p.

HELSINKI DECLARATION: BIOETHICAL ISSUES, CLINICAL RIGHTS OF HUMANS, PRINCIPLES OF RESEARCH ON HUMANS AND NATURE OF HUMAN EXPERIMENTATION. June 2002. Cloth is 57.50, ISBN 0-7883-2830-1; Pb is 47.50, ISBN 0-7883-2831-X.

HOT FLASHES: Index of New Information and Guide-Book for Consumers, Reference and Research. June 2002. Cloth $ 57.50, ISBN 0-7883-2730-5; Pb is 47.50, ISBN 0-7883-2731-3. American Health Research Institute. 160p.

WEST NILE FEVER–Outbreaks and Conditions in the U.S. and Elsewhere: Index of New Information and Guide-Book for Reference, Research & Clinical Uses. September 2002. Cloth $ 57.50, ISBN 0-7883-2742-9; PB 47.50 ISBN 0-7883-2743-7.

HOW CAN ANYONE IMPROVE THE HEALTH OF ALL PEOPLE? BY ONE SIMPLE MANEUVER: TAKE THE POLITICS OUT OF RESEARCH PROJECTS !

CANCER ENCYCLOPEDIA --Collections of Anti-Cancer and Anti-Carcinogenic Agents, chemicals, drugs and substances: Index of New Information and Guide-Book for Consumers, Reference and Research. January 2002. Volumes are available as a set or as separate volumes in Hardcover or Paperback.

20 Volume set. Hardcover: 0-7883-2650-3: $ 1310.00. Approx 3600+ pages. (Paperback listings follow on the next page)

Volume 1   (1969-1979) Cloth, 65.50: ISBN 0-7883-2652-X. 180p.
Volume 2   (1980-1985) Cloth, 65.50: ISBN 0-7883-2654-6. 180p.
Volume 3   (1986-1988) Cloth, 65.50: ISBn 0-7883-2656-2. 180p.
Volume 4   (1989-1991) Cloth, 65.50: ISBN 0-7883-2658-9. 180p.
Volume 5   (1992)   Cloth, 65.50: ISBN 0-7883-2660-0. 180p.
Volume 6   (1993)   Cloth, 65.50: ISBN 0-7883-2662-7. 180p.
Volume 7   (1994)   Cloth, 65.50: ISBN 0-7883-2664-3. 180p.
Volume 8   (1995A)   Cloth, 65.50: ISBN 0-7883-2666-X. 180p.
Volume 9   (1995B)   Cloth, 65-50: ISBN 0-7883-2668-6. 180p.
Volume 10 (1996A)   Cloth, 65-50: ISBN 0-7883-2670-8. 180p.
Volume 11 (1996B)   Cloth, 65.50: ISBN 0-7883-2672-4. 180p.
Volume 12 (1997A)   Cloth, 65.50: ISBN 0-7883-2674-0. 180p.
Volume 13 (1997B)   Cloth, 65.50: ISBN 0-7883-2676-7. 180p.
Volume 14 (1998A)   Cloth, 65.50: ISBN 0-7883-2678-3. 180p.
Volume 15 (1998B)   Cloth, 65.50: ISBN 0-7883-2680-5. 180p.
Volume 16 (1999A)   Cloth, 65.50: ISBN 0-7883-2682-1. 180p.
Volume 17 (1999B)   Cloth, 65.50: ISBN 0-7883-2684-8. 180p.
Volume 18 (2000A)   Cloth, 65.50: ISBN 0-7883-2686-4. 180p.
Volume 19 (2000B)   Cloth, 65.50: ISBN 0-7883-2688-0. 180p.
Volume 20 (2000C)   Cloth, 65.50: ISBN 0-7883-2690-2. 180p.
20 Volume Set: Hardcover: 0-7883-2650-3: $ 1310.00 Approx 3600+ pages. Paperback volumes, price and ISBN follow on the next page.

Collective Bargaining, Labor Unions and Negotiations: Index of New Information for Analysis, Reference and Research. May 2002. Cloth $ 57.50, ISBN 0-7883-2640-6; Pb is $ 47.50, ISBN 0-7883-2641-4. Science & Life Consultants Asn. 180p.

MANDATORY TESTING OF SUBSTANCE ABUSE: INDEX OF NEW INFORMATION AND GUIDE-BOOK FOR REFERENCE AND RESEARCH. 2nd Edition Cloth Cloth $65.00, ISBN 0-7883-2782-6; Pb is $47.50, ISBN 0-7883-2783-6. S & L Consultants.

POLICE –Health, Risks, Shift Work, Attitudes and Brutality Force: Index of New information. 2nd Revision, New. Cloth $61.00, ISBN is 0-7884-2890-5; PB is $51.00, ISBN is 0-7883-2891-3. Dr. Walter E. Schultz. 180p.

BIBLIOGRAPHIC INFORMATION FOR ALL NATIONS

8

RESEARCH AND PROGRESS FOR ALL MANKIND

NEW REFERENCE BOOKS AND RESEARCH INDEXES

WORLD COMMERCIALISM IS INVOLVED IN WORLD-WIDE CANCER EPIDEMICS

CANCER ENCYCLOPEDIA -Collections of Anti-Cancer & Anti-Carcinogenic
Agents, Chemicals, Drugs and Substances:
Index of New Information and Guide-Book for
Consumers, Reference and Research. January
2002. Approx 3600 pages. Dr. John C. Bartone.

PAPERBACK VOLUMES: AVAILABLE AS SET OR AS INDIVIDUAL VOLUMES:
**Publication Date: January 2002.
20 Volume set: Paperback: ISBN 0-7883-2651-1: $ 1110.00; Approx 3600 pages.

Volume 1 (1966-1979) Paperback, 55.50: ISBN 0-7883-2653-8. 180p.
Volume 2 (1980-1985) Paperback, 55.50: ISBN 0-7883-2655-4. 180p.
Volume 3 (1986-1988) Paperback, 55.50: ISBN 0-7883-2657-0. 180p.
Volume 4 (1989-1991) Paperback, 55.50: ISBN 0-7883-2659-7. 180p.
Volume 5 (1992)   Paperback, 55.50: ISBN 0-7883-2661-9. 180p.
Volume 6 (1993)   Paperback, 55.50: ISBN 0-7883-2663-5. 180p.
Volume 7 (1994)   Paperback, 55.50: ISBN 0-7883-2665-1. 180p.
Volume 8 (1995A)   Paperback, 55.50: ISBN 0-7883-2667-8. 180p.
Volume 9 (1885B)   Paperback, 55.50: ISBN 0-7885-2669-4. 180p.
Volume 10 (1996A)   Paperback, 55.50: ISBN 0-7883-2671-6. 180p.
Volume 11 (1996B)   Paperback, 55.50: ISBN 0-7883-2673-2. 180p.
Volume 12 (1997A)   Paperback, 55.50: ISBN 0-7883-2675-9. 180p.
Volume 13 (1997B)   Paperback, 55.50: ISBN 0-7883-2677-5. 180p.
Volume 14 (1998A)   Paperback, 55.50: ISBN 0-7883-2679-1. 180p.
Volume 15 (1998B)   Paperback, 55.50: ISBN 0-7883-2681-3. 180p.
Volume 16 (1999A)   Paperback, 55.50: ISBN 0-7883-2683-X. 180p.
Volume 17 (1999B)   Paperback, 55.50: ISBN 0-7883-2685-6. 180p.
Volume 18 (2000A)   Paperback, 55.50: ISBN 0-7883-2687-2. 180p.
Volume 19 (2000B)   Paperback, 55.50: ISBN 0-7883-2689-9. 180p.
Volume 20 (2000C)   Paperback, 55.50: ISBN 0-7883-2691-0. 180p.

Pneumonia —Medical Subject Analysis, Reference and Research Guide-Book.
January 2002. Cloth $57.50, ISBN 0-7883-2804-2; Pb is $47.50,
ISBN 0-7883-2805-0 Dr. Dominic Stannic. 180p.

Pollutant Materials —Index of New Information and Guide-Book for Consumers,
Reference & Research. January 2002. Cloth $57.50, ISBN 0-7883-
2572-8; Pb is $47.50, ISBN 0-7883-2573-4. Dr. Claudia Franconio.

NEURO-TOXINS —Index of New Information and Research Reference Bible.
April 2001. Cloth $57.50, ISBN 0-7883-2452-7; PB is 47.50, ISBN
0-7883-2453-5. R & D Division. 180p.

FAX ORDERS TO: (703) 642-5966: OPEN 24 HOURS A DAY X 7 DAYS A WEEK.

RESEARCH AND PROGRESS FOR ALL MANKIND

NEW REFERENCE BOOKS AND RESEARCH INDEXES

NEGLECT OF RESEARCH PROGRESS INCREASES CRIME, DISEASE & POVERTY

EMBRYO RESEARCH IN TODAY'S WORLD: Index of New Information and Guide-Book for Consumers, Reference and Research. January 2002. Cloth is $57.50, ISBN 0-7883-2700-3; PB is $47.50, ISBN 0-7883-2701-1. Dr. Joy W. Rader. 180p.

ORGAN DONATIONS OF HUMANS: index of New Information and Guide-Book for Consumers, Reference and Research. January 2002. Cloth is $57.50, ISBN 0-7883-2574-4; Pb is $47.50, ISBN 0-7883-2575-2. Dr. Susan Morganstein. 180p.

SEX, DYSFUNCTIONS AND PARAPHILIAS: Index of New Information and Guide-Book for Consumers, Reference and Research. January 2002. Cloth is $57.50 ISBN 0-7883-2578-7; PB is $47.50, ISBN 0-7883-2579-5. Dr. Peter J Nelson. 180p.

SOCCER –REPORT FOR ATHLETES, COACHES AND CONSUMERS; Index of New Information and Guide-Book for Consumers, Reference and Research. January 2002. Cloth is $57.50, ISBN 0-7883-2582-5; Pb is $47.50, ISBN 0-7883-2583-3. Dr. Jerry J. Reeder. 180p.

COMPUTER NETWORKS IN THE HEALTH PROFESSIONS; Index of New Information and Guide-Book for Consumers, Reference and Research. January 2002. Cloth $57.50, ISBN 0-7883-2596-5; Pb is 47.50, ISBN 0-7883-2597-3. Dr. Fred G. Zollinger. 180p.

CHEMICAL WARFARE; Index of New information and Guide-Book for Consumers, Reference and Research. January 2002. Cloth $57.50, ISBN 0-7883-2598-1; Pb is $47.50, ISBN 0-7883-2599-X. Dr. Patrick W. Zacherie.

INFANT FOOD: Index of New Information and Guide-Book for Consumers, Reference and Research. February 2002. Cloth $57.50, ISBN 0-7883-2624-4; Pb is $47.50, ISBN 0-7883-2625-2. Dr. Alberta G. Torres.

SEX AND ORGASM; index of New Information and Guide-Book for Consumers, Reference and Research. February 2002. Cloth $57.50, ISBN 0-7883-2748-8; Pb is $47.50, ISBN 0-7883-2749-6. Dr. Peter J. Nelson.

COMPUTERS –USE AND DEVELOPMENT FOR HEALTH SCIENTISTS; Index of New Information and Guide-Book for Consumers, Reference and Research. February 2002. Cloth $57.50, ISBN 0-7883-2738-0; Pb is 47.50, ISBN 0-7883-2739-9. Dr. Fred D. Zollinger. 180p.

Breast CANCER; Index of New Information and Guide-Book for Consumers, Reference and Research. January 2002. Cloth $57.50, ISBN 0-7883-2606-6; Pb is $47.50, ISBN 0-7883-2607-4. Dr. Karia Marvis Verbeke.

FAX ORDERS TO: (703) 642-5966: OPEN 24 HOURS A DAY X 7 DAYS A WEEK.

RESEARCH AND PROGRESS FOR ALL MANKIND

NEW REFERENCE BOOKS AND RESEARCH INDEXES

RICH NATIONS PROFIT THE MOST FROM ALL FORMS OF RESEARCH

BIOLOGY OF WARFARE: Index of New Information and Guide-Book for Consumers, Reference and Research. January 2002. Cloth $57.50, ISBN 0-7883-2638-4; Pb is $47.50, ISBN 0-7883-2639-2. Dr. G. Schiff.

POLLUTANT MATERIALS: Index of New Information and Guide-Book for Consumers, Reference and Research. January 2002. Cloth $57.50, ISBN 0-7883-2572-8; Pb is 47.50, ISBN 0-7883-2573-4. Dr. Claudia J. Franconio. 180p.

WESCHSLER SCALES; Index of New Information and Guide-Book for Consumers, Reference and Research. January 2002. Cloth $57.50, ISBN 0-7883-2718-6; Pb is $47.50, ISBN 0-7883-2719-4. Dr. William R. Ellington. 180p.

BETA-CAROTENE: Index of New Information and Guide-Book for Consumers, Reference and Research. January 2002. Cloth $57.50, ISBN 0-7883-2590-6; Pb is $47.50, ISBN 0-7883=2591-4. Dr. Jimmie C. Chen. 180p.

Menstruation Disturbances: Index of New Information and Guide-Book for Consumers, Reference and Research. March 2002. Cloth, 57.50:ISBN 0-7883-2528-0; PB is ISBN 0-7883-2529-9. 175p. Dr. Estelle S. Dornato.

HISTORIC NOTE

REFERENCE BOOKS, NEW OR OLD, NEVER DIE OR BECOME OBSOLETE FOR THEY TELL OF THE PROGRESS OF THE PRESENT ERA, YIELD MANY LANDMARKS OF THE PAST AND SERVE AS WISE GUIDE-POSTS TO THE FUTURE OF ALL MANKIND.

Dr. Felix-Anthony Bertone, Ph.D.
Rome, 1906

NEW REFERENCE BOOKS & RESEARCH INDEXES

WITHOUT RESEARCH OUR LIFE-SPAN
WOULD BE LESS
THAN 40 YEARS!

ACETAMINOPHEN: INDEX
ETHYLENE: INDEX
ACIDOSIS: INDEX
ACUPUNCTURE: INDEX
ACYCLOVIR: INDEX
ADOLESCENT BEHAVIOR: INDEX
ADOLESCENT PSYCHOLOGY: INDEX
ADVERSE EFFECTS OF AIR POLLUTANTS: INDEX
ADVERSE EFFECTS OF ASPIRIN: INDEX
ADVERSE EFFECTS OF LITHIUM: INDEX

ADVERSE EFFECTS OF RADIOTHERAPY: INDEX
ADVERTISING & MEDICINE: GUIDEBOOK INDEX
AEROSPACE MEDICINE: INDEX
AGED & THE ELDERLY: INDEX
AGGRESSION: INDEX
AIR ANALYSIS FOR HEALTH & DANGERS AT HOME:
AIR POLLUTANTS: INDEX
AIR POLLUTION FUNGUS & MOLDS IN HOMES, ET
AIRCRAFTS & AIR TRANSPORT IN COMMERCE & MED:

ALCOHOL DRINKiNG: INDEX
ALKALOSIS: INDEX
ALLERGY & IMMUNOLOGY: INDEX
ALUMINUM: INDEX
ALZHEIMER'S DISEASE: INDEX
AMBULATORY CARE: INDEX
ANATOMY & HEALTH SCIENCE: INDEX
ANIMAL BEHAVIOR: INDEX
ANIMAL COMMUNICATIONS: INDEX
ANIMAL HUSBANDRY: INDEX

ANIMAL PHYSIOLOGY: INDEX
ANIMAL SOCIAL BEHAVIOR: INDEX
ANIMAL TESTING ALTERNATIVES
ANIMAL WELFARE: INDEX
ANIMALS IN MEDICINE & RESEARCH
ANIMALS IN WILDLIFE: INDEX
ANTHROPOLOGY OF MINORITY GROUPS
ANTI-OXIDANTS: INDEX
ANTI-OXIDANTS: EFFECTS ON LONGEVITY

NEW REFERENCE BOOKS & RESEARCH INDEXES

NEW RESEARCH LEADS TO PROGRESS
AND
HEALTH IMPROVEMENTS FOR YOU....

ANTI-OXIDANTS & TOXICITY RESEARCH
ANTIBIOTICS & ADVERSE EFFECTS
ANXIETY -PREVENTION & CONTROL
ANXIETY DISORDERS
APTITUDE TESTS
ARM INJURIES

ARTIFICIAL INTELLIGENCE
ASBESTOS & ASBESTOSIS
ASPIRIN -REPORTS OF HARMFUL EFFECTS
ATHEROSCLEROSIS: INDEX OF REVIEWS
ATHEROSCLEROSIS & ATHERECTOMY

ATHLETIC INJURIES: GUIDEBOOK
ATTEMPTED SUICIDE: GUIDEBOOK
ATTITUDE & ATTITUDES: INDEX
ATTITUDES TO DEATH & DYING
AUDIO-VISUAL AIDS IN HEALTH BIOLOGY
AUTOMATIC DATA TECHNOLOGY
AUTOMATION & AUTOANALYSIS IN MED
AUTO ACCIDENTS, PREVENTION & CONTROL
AUTO EXHAUST IN HEALTH & DISEASE

BACK PAIN & SPINAL PROBLEMS
BACTERIA: INDEX OF REVIEWS
BACTERIAL INFECTIONS
BARTONE'S GUIDEBOOK TO BIOL WARFARE
BARTONELLA INFECTIONS
BEHAVIOR & MOTIVATION
BEHAVIOR IN MIND & BODY BY CHOICE
BEHAVIORAL SCIENCES
BENZENE

BETA-CAROTENE & CAROTENOIDS
BEVERAGES, DRINKS & JUICES
BIBLE QUOTATIONS MADE HUMOROUS
BIBLES: INDEX OF MODERN INFORMATION
BIBLIOGRAPHY & DOCUMENTATION IN HEALTH
BIBLIOGRAPHY PUBLICATIONS
BIO-ETHICS: INDEX
BIOLOGICAL PRODUCTS & ACTIONS
BIOLOGY IN THE HEALTH SCIENCES

NEW REFERENCE BOOKS & RESEARCH INDEXES

REFERENCE BOOKS & INDEXES ARE PIONEERS
AND LEAD YOU
INTO NEW UNKNOWN VISTAS
FOR GREATER WEALTH,
WISDOM AND HEALTH

BIOLOGY OF ALLIGATORS & CROCODILES
BIOLOGY OF COCKROACHES: INDEX
BIOLOGY OF FLEAS: INDEX
BIOLOGY OF SURVIVAL: HUMAN, ANIMAL LIFE
BIOMEDICAL ENGINEERING
BIORHYTHMS, BIOLOGICAL CLOCKS & PERIODICITY
BIOSENSORS & TECHNICAL MED
BIOTECHNOLOGY
BIRTH INJURIES

BLACKS & THE NEGROID RACE
BLACKS & THEIR BIO-MEDICAL HISTORY
BLACKS--STATUS & PROGRESS
BLACKS--THEIR PSYCHOLOGY & BEHAVIOR

BLINDNESS
BLOOD PRESSURE & DRUG EFFECTS
BLOOD SUBSTITUTES & THER USES
BRAIN INJURIES
BRAIN METABOLIC DISEASES
BREAST CANCERS, CHEMICALLY INDUCED
BREATH TESTS IN HEALTH, SCIENCE & MEDICINE
BUFOTENIN (DIMETHYLSEROTONIN)
BURNS-THERAPY & PSYCHOLOGY

BUTTER--ANALYSIS, COMPOSITION, USES, FLAVOR
CAESARIAN SECTION & BIRTH FACTORS
CAFFEINE: INDEX

CANCER & CARCINOGENS IN HOME, WORK, ET
CANCER AND ITS CAUSES
CANCER & IT PSYCHOLOGICAL INFLUENCES
CANCER & PRECANCEROUS CONDITIONS
CANCER--RESEARCH ON CAUSES
CANCER PREVENTION & CONTROL
CANCER THERAPY--METHODS, TREATMENT, ET
CANCER VARIATIONS & MORTALITY
CANCERS--BY EXPERIMENTS, CHEM PRODUCTS
CANCERS PRODUCED BY RADIATION
CANNABIS (MARIJUANA)

CARCINOGENS

NEW REFERENCE BOOKS & RESEARCH INDEXES

NEW INFORMATION PROLONGS LIFE -
AND
SOMETIMES HAPPINESS TOO!

CARDIOPULMONARY BYPASS
CARPAL TUNNEL SYNDROME-CAUSES, TREATMENT
CAT DISEASES & VET MED
CELL NEOPLASTIC TRANSFORMATION
CEREALS, GRAIN, MALT & MILLET
CHARITIES, GOOD WILL & DIVINE GIVING

CHEMICAL INDUCTION, NEW TUMORS, CANCER
CHILD ABUSE: REFERENCE GUIDE & INDEX
CHILD ABUSE II: REFERENCE GUIDE & INDEX
CHILD PLAY & PLAYTHINGS: INDEX
CHILD WELFARE & FOSTER HOME CARE
CHILDREN'S DAILY VERSES FOR FUN & PLAY
CHIN AND MANDIBLE
CHIROPRACTIC PRACTICE-METHODS, TRENDS
CHRISTIANITY: INDEX OF MODERN INFO
CHROMIUM IN HEALTH, DISEASE & INDUSTRY

CIRCUMCISION: PROS AND
CIVIL DEFENSE IN WAR & PEACE
CIVIL RIGHTS
CLOTHING, HEALTH, HAZARD, STYLES, IMAGE PSYC
COCAINE & ITS DAMAGING INFLUENCES
COMMUNICABLE DISEASES
COMMUNICATION-PERSUASIVE, MASTER-MIND, PROPAGANDA
COMMUNICATION IN MED & PSYCHOLOGY
COMMUNISM: INDEX

COMPETITIVE BEHAVIOR

COMPUTER ADVANCEMENTS IN HEALTH SCIENCE
COMPUTER ASSISTED INSTRUCTION IN HS
COMPUTER COMMUNICATION NETWORKS
COMPUTER SCIEBCE & INFORMATICS IN MEDICINE
COMPUTER SCIENCE IN HEALTH SCIENCE
COMPUTER ASSISTED DIAGNOSIS
COMPUTER ASSISTED INSTRUCTION & EDUCATION
CONSERVATION

CONSUMER & PATIENT SATISFACTION
CONSUMER & PUBLIC DISCLOSURE OF CONDOMS
CONSUMER ATTITUDES & WISH OF HEALTH CARE

NEW REFERENCE BOOKS & RESEARCH INDEXES

AUTHORS (SCIENTISTS) PRODUCE RESEARCH
AND
NEW PRODUCTS
FOR BETTER LIFE, NOW AND FUTURE LIVING

CONSUMER CAR CARE FOR WISE, POOR & HELPLESS
CONSUMER INDEX BOOK: COCAINE & DANGER
CONSUMER INDEX: HAZARD SUBSTANCE IN YOUR LIFE
CONSUMER INDEX ABOUT HIV, AIDS & TREATMENTS
CONSUMER INDEX ABOUT INFORMED CONSENT
CONSUMERS' ATTITUDES TO HEALTH CARE
CONSUMER'S' INDEX ABOUT DIAGNOSTIC ERRORS
CONSUMER'S' DATA BOOK OF ACTIVITIES, INVESTIG, ORG

CONSUMERS' INDEX: WHAT'S GOING ON IN LIFE, ET
CONSUMERS' INDEX ABOUT ABORTION, TODAY'S WORLD
CONSUMERS' INDEX ABOUT ADOLESCENT BEHAVIOR
CONSUMERS' INDEX ABOUT AUTO ACCIDENTS
CONSUMERS' INDEX ABOUT CIVIL RIGHTS

CONSUMERS' INDEX ABOUT COSMETICS GOOD & BAD
CONSUMERS' INDEX ABOUT CRIME PREVENTION
CONSUMERS' INDEX ABOUT CRIME TODAY IN U.S.A.
CONSUMERS' INDEX ABOUT EXERCISE
CONSUMER'S INDEX ABOUT FOOD, DIET & CANCER
CONSUMERS' INDEX ABOUT HUMAN RIGHTS

CONSUMERS' INDEX ABOUT HYPNOSIS
CONSUMERS' INDEX ABOUT ILLNESS & DISEASE BY JOBS
CONSUMERS' INDEX ABOUT JUVENILE DELINQUENCY
CONSUMERS' INDEX LOVE AND LIBIDO

CONSUMERS' INDEX ABOUT MAGIC & SUPERSTITIONS
CONSUMERS' INDEX ABOUT MARRIAGE
CONSUMERS' INDEX ABOUT MASSAGE
CONSUMERS' INDEX ABOUT NUTRITION
CONSUMERS' INDEX ABOUT RELAXATION & METHODS

CONSUMERS' INDEX ABOUT RIGHTS TO MED TREATMENT
CONSUMERS' INDEX ABOUT SEX & BISEXUALITY
CONSUMERS' INDEX ABOUT SEX COUNSELING & DISEASE
CONSUMERS' INDEX ABOUT SPORTS

CONSUMERS' INDEX ABOUT STRESS, DISTRESS & TRMT
CONSUMERS' INDEX ABOUT HEALTH BENEFITS OF GARLIC
CONSUMERS' INDEX ABOUT .....DEATH

NEW REFERENCE BOOKS & RESEARCH INDEXES

NATIONS OR PEOPLE WITHOUT RESEARCH PROGRESS BECOME EASY VICTIMS OF TIME, ROT AND SICK HEALTH

CONSUMERS' INDEX ABOUT MEDICAL MALPRACTICE
CONSUMERS' RIGHTS AS ARMED CITIZENS
CONSUMERS' INDEX: WHAT'S GOING ON IN LIFE, ET
CONSUMERS' INDEX ABOUT ABORTION

CONTRACEPTION & FAMILY PLANNING
CORONARY DISEASE

COSMETICS & BEAUTY CULTURE
COSMETICS & HEALTH
COTTON --IN HEALTH, WORK & INDUSTRY
COUNSELING-GUIDE, INTERVENTION, SKILLS, MGT, SEX

CRIME
CRIME & CRIMINAL NOTIONS
CRIME & CRIMINAL PSYCHOLOGY

CRIME AND RIOT CONTROL
CRIME ANALYSIS-WITH MED, FORENSIC, POLITICS
CRIME PREVENTION AND CONTROL
CRIME RESEARCH INDEX

CRIMINAL PSYCHOLOGY
CRISIS INTERVENTION
CURRICULUMS IN HEALTH SCIENCES
CYSTIC FIBROSIS
DEATH
DEATH & POST CHANGES, NORM & MYSTERIOUS
DECISION MAKING IN HEALTH
DELIVERY OF HEALTH CARE & INTL MED
DENTAL CARE & HEALTH FACTORS

DENTAL PRACTICE & RESEARCH
DENTISTRY IN INDUSTRY
DENTISTRY, PATIENTS & DENTISTS

DEODORANTS
DEPRESSION
DEVELOPING COUNTRIES
DIAGNOSIS
DIAGNOSIS & COMPUTERS

NEW REFERENCE BOOKS & RESEARCH INDEXES.

RESEARCH PATHWAYS ARE SECRET ROADS TO DRIVE TO UTOPIA FOR EVERYONE.

DIAGNOSIS OF DEPRESSIVE DISORDERS
DIAGNOSIS OF MENTAL DISORDERS
DIAGNOSTIC ERRORS IN MEDICINE
DIAGNOSTIC TESTS

DIET -IN LIFE, FOOD, OLD AGE & RESEARCH
DIET -INVESTIGATIONS, RESEARCH, RESULTS
DIETARY FIBER
DIETARY FIBER, CALORIES AND CANCER

DIETARY MINERALS & DANGEROUS INFLUENCE

DIETHEL SULFOXIDE (DMSO)

DIOXINS & AGENT ORANGE

DIRECTORIES, ASSOCIATIONS, SOCIETIES
DIRECTORY, NEW REVIEWS: ALCOHOLISM
DIRECTORY, REVIEWS, AMBULATORY SURGERY
DIRECTORY, REVIEWS, ANTI-CANCER AGENTS
DIRECTORY, REVIEWS OF ANTIBIOTICS
DIRECTORY, REVIEWS OF ANTIGENS OF CANCER
DIRECTORY, REVIEWS OF BIOPSY
DIRECTORY, REVIEWS OF CARCINOGENS

DIRECTORY, REVIEWS, CELL MEMBRANES
DIRECTORY, REVIEWS: CERVIX NEOPLASMS
DIRECTORY, REVIEWS OF COENZYMES
DIRECTORY, REVIEWS OF CONTRACEPTION

DIRECTORY, REVIEWS OF CYSTIC FIBROSIS
DIRECTORY, REVIEWS OF DIABETES MELLITUS
DIRECTORY, REVIEWS OF DIETS

DIRECTORY, REVIEWS OF DOMESTIC ANIMALS
DIRECTORY, REVIEWS OF ECOLOGY
DIRECTORY, REVIEWS OF HOMEOSTASIS
DIRECTORY, REVIEWS: IMMUNOGLOBULINS
DIRECTORY, REVIEWS OF IMMUNOTHERAPY

DIRECTORY, REVIEWS OF INTELLIGENCE

NEW REFERENCE BOOKS & RESEARCH INDEXES

RESEARCH IS THE BEATING HEART -
AND BLOOD-
OF PROGRESS
AGAINST ALL FORMS OF DECAY.

DIR ECTORY, REVIEWS OF LEUKOCYTES
DIRECTORY, REVIEWS OF MALARIA
DIRECTORY, REVIEWS OF MENTAL DISORDERS
DIRECTORY, REVIEWS OF MINERAL OIL
DIRECTORY, REVIEWS, NEUROTRANS RECEPT
DIRECTORY, REVIEWS OF PHAGOCYTES
DIRECTORY, REVIEWS OF PHYLOGENY
DIRECTORY, REVIEWS, POST-SURGERY COMPLICATIONS
DIRECTORY, REVIEWS: RHEUMATIC DISEASES
DIRECTORY, REVIEWS, SUDDEN CARDIAC DEATHS

DIRECTORY, REVIEWS: TUMOR NECROSIS FACTOR
DIRECTORY, REVIEWS OF XENOBIOTICS
DISABILITY EVALUATION
DISASTERS & DISASTER PLANNING
DISEASE SUSCEPTIBILITY
DISINFECTION & STERILIZATION

DIVORCE & DIVORCE FACTORS
DNA & RECOMBINANTS

DNA FINGER-PRINTING
DOG DISEASES

DREAMS

DRUG ADDICTION, SUBSTANCE ABUSE & DEPENDENCE
DRUG EFFECTS ON MEMORY
DRUG EFFECTS ON MENTAL PROCESSES
DRUG EFFECTS ON THE FETUS
DRUG THERAPY FACTORS & ADVERSE EFFECTS
DRUG THERAPY IN HEALTH, MED & DISEASE
DRUG WITHDRAWAL SYMPTOMS
DRUGS IN ALL PHASES OF LIFE & MED

DRUGS & PSYCHOLOGICAL EFFECT ON BEHAV
DUST & PNEUMOCONIOSIS
DYSLEXIA
EDEMA RESEARCH

EDUCATION & ITS MEASUREMENT

NEW REFERENCE BOOKS & RESEARCH INDEXES

MUCH GRADUATE RESEARCH OF STUDENTS
IS NEVER PUBLISHED
AND
MADE AVAILABLE
TO HELP WORLD PROGRESS:
WHY NOT, AND WHO IS AT FAULT?

EDUCATIONAL MEASUREMENT
EFFICIENCY & PERFORMANCE
ELECTRIC INJURIES INCLUDING LIGHTNING
ELECTRONIC MAIL & OFFICE AUTOMATION

ELECTRONICS IN HEALTH SCIENCES
EMOTIONS AND MOODS

EMPLOYMENT, WORK & HEALTH
ENDOCRINOLOGY
ENERGY-GENERATING RESOURCES
EPILEPSY
EPILEPSY: NEW REVIEWS
ESTROGEN DEFICIENCY & DEPRIVATION
ESTROGENS

EUGENICS
EUTHANASIA

EVOLUTION & LIFE SCIENCES

EXERCISE BY WALKING
EXERCISE TESTS & SPORTS MEDICINE
EXERCISE THERAPY
EXERTION
EXPERT TESTIMONY IN MED, LAW, ETC
EYE INJURIES

FACIAL EXPRESSIONS, ANATOMY, ANALYSIS
FACIAL INJURIES I
FAMILY PRACTICE

FAMILY THERAPY
FEAR AND PANIC
FEARS AND PHOBIAS
FEMALE GENITAL DISEASES
FETAL DEVELOPMENT
FETAL MONITORING
FIBER OPTICS
FINGER INJURIES

FIREARMS & GUNSHOT WOUNDS

NEW REFERENCE BOOKS & RESEARCH INDEXES

TO INNOVATE --IS TO MAKE CHANGES -
IT IS A "NEW" AND EASY METHOD
TO PROMOTE RESEARCH
AND
INCREASE A NATION'S WEALTH AND HEALTH

FIRES
FIRST AID
FIRST AID & EMERGENCIES

FISH OILS IN HEALTH & DISEASE
FISHES (TILAPIA)
FLOWMETERS (RHEOLOGY)
FLUOXETINE (PROZAC, ET)

FOOD & DIET: HARMFUL REPORTS, ILL, CANCER
FOOD & ITS DANGEROUS INGREDIENTS
FOOD ADDITIVES
FOOD ADDITIVES: HARMFUL REACTIONS, ETC
FOOD--CALORIE INTAKE & EFFECTS

FOOD COLORING AGENTS & TOXICITY
FOOD CONTAMINATION
FOOD DISPENSERS & VENDING MACHINES
FOOD HABITS AND CUSTOMS
FOOD IRRADIATION
FOOD MANIA AND OVER-EATING
FOOD SWEETENERS -ASPARTAME & ADVERSE R
FOOD VALUES & BIOAVAILABILITY

FOOT CARE & RESEARCH

FOOTBALL
FORECASTING
FOUNDATIONS: GOALS & ROLES
FRACTURES

FRAUD, MALPRACTICE, PRETENSE, DECEPTION
FUTUROLOGY
GARLIC: MEDICAL & HEALTH QUALITIES
GASOLINE
GASTRO-INTESTINAL DISEASES

GENEALOGY & RELATIVE FACTORS
GENETIC ENGINEERING & CELL INTERVENTION
GENETIC SCREENING
GENETIC TOXICITY TESTS
GENOME BIOLOGY

NEW REFERENCE BOOKS & RESEARCH INDEXES

RESEARCH IS THE MOST UN-DEVELOPED THEME IN ALL NATIONS --
WHAT A TRAGEDY!

GERIATRICS & MEDICINE

GINSENG -IN LIFE & HEALTH
GLASS & GLASSOIDS

GLAUCOMA

GOLD -STUDIES & USES
GOVERNMENTS & AGENCIES: ACTIVITIES & INFORMATION
GROWTH SUBSTANCES
GUIDEBOOK & REF: MED COMPUTERS

GUNS & FIREARMS: MEDICAL, PSYCHOLOGIC, LEGAL IML
GUNS, THE CONSUMER & ANTI-GUN COHORTS
GUNS, FIREARMS, CRIME & CONTROVERSY
GUNS, THE N.R.A. & CONSUMERS ARMED
GUNSHOT WOUNDS IN CRIME & MED
GYMNASTICS & VARIATIONS

HAIR ANALYSIS

HAND INJURIES
HANDICAPPED & THE DISABLED

HAZARDOUS SUBSTANCES IN HEALTH, BEHAV, INDUSTRY

HEAD & NECK CANCERS
HEAD INJURIES

HEALTH & BIO-SCIENCE AWARDS, PRIZES
HEALTH & LIFE HAZARDS
HEALTH & MED ASPECTS: CHEM INDUSTRIES
HEALTH & MED DIAGNOSTIC ERRORS: THERAPY & TREAT
HEALTH -DANGERS, RISKS AND ASSESSMENTS
HEALTH CARE FINANCING IN U.S.

HEALTH CARE REFORM: SPECIFICS, ECONOMICS, LEGISLAT

HEALTH CARE SERVICES IN PRISONS
HEALTH DANGERS IN OUR DRINKING WATER
HEALTH DOCTORS WITH IMPAIRMENTS, AIDS, ETC
HEALTH DOCTORS; VIEWS, WRITINGS, RIGHTS, ET
HEALTH EDUCATION

NEW REFERENCE BOOKS & RESEARCH INDEXES

RESEARCH REQUIRES A WELL-EDUCATED MIND AND SOMEONE WITH SOME CURIOSITY.

****ALL CITIZENS MUST TEACH POLITICIANS THE IMPORTANCE OF RESEARCH FOR ALL PEOPLE

HEALTH HAZARDS, SKIN PROBLEMS BY WORK
HEALTH HAZARDS IN OCCUPATIONS

HEALTH INSURANCE FOR AGED & DISABLED: T18
HEALTH MAINTAIN ORG (HM0)
HEALTH POLICY FOR HIV INFECTION & AIDS
HEALTH POLICY WITH PLANS, PRIORITIES, P & P
HEALTH PRIORITIES IN THE U.S.A.
HEALTH PROGRAMS: SCOPE, STRAT,CRITIC & PRAC
HEALTH PROMOTION
HEALTH PROTECTION & IMPROVEMENTS BY ADVICE, ET
HEALTH RESEARCH

HEALTH RESORTS & MEDICINE
HEALTH SCIENCE DOCUMENTATIONS
HEALTH SCIENCES RESEARCH I
HEALTH SCIENTISTS BIBLE OF BIBLIOGRAPHY
HEALTH SCIENTISTS BIBLE OF BIBLIOGRAPHY

HEALTH STATUS INDICATORS
HEARING & HEARING DISORDERS
HEART ATTACKS & REHABILITATION
HEART ATTACKS: REAL, IMAGINED, SUSPICIOUS
HEART FUNCTION TESTS
HEART INJURIES
HEMODYNAMICS: DIRECTORY & REVIEWS INDEX

HEMORRHOIDS

HEPATITIS C: DIRECTORY & REVIEWS INDEX
HERNIA -SIMPLE & COMPLEX
HERPES GENITALIS

HISTORY OF MEDICINE
HISTORY OF PRISONS
HISTORY OF WAR
HIV TRACING & TRANSMISSION: WORK, SPORTS, ETC
HOLOCAUST

NEW REFERENCE BOOKS & RESEARCH INDEXES

RESEARCH HELPS ALL BABIES
TO A HEALTHY
BIRTH AND A THRIVING CHILDHOOD.

HOME CARE SERVICES
HOMELESS & STREET PEOPLE

HOMEOPATHY
HOMICIDE
HOMOSEXUALITY
HORMONE PHYSIOLOGY
HORMONES

HORSES
HOSPICE & TERMINAL CARE
HOSPITAL ECONOMICS

HOSPITAL INFECTIONS & PATIENTS
HOSPITAL INFECTIONS: PREVENTION & CONTROL
HOSPITALIZATION
HOSTILITY CHARACTERISTICS & BEHAV
HOTLINES: PURPOSE, SERV & NEEDS

HUMAN ABNORMALITIES CAUSED BY CHEM, DRUGS, ETC
HUMAN ABORTION
HUMAN BEHAVIOR & REACTIONS TO LIVING
HUMAN BEHAVIOR & SOCIAL CONTROL MANAGEMENT

HUMAN BEHAVIOR: ANALYSIS, THERAPY, TREATMENTS
HUMAN CONCEPTS OF LIFE, LOVE, WORK
HUMAN DESIRES & EXPECTATIONS OF FUTURE
HUMAN EXPERIMENTATION

HUMAN HEMORRHOIDS

HUMAN LIFE EXPECTANCY:EXPERIEN & ANAL
HUMAN LIVING AND HOW LIFE-EVENTS INFLUEN
HUMAN LONGEVITY: ANAL, INFLUENCE, RISKS, ETC
HUMAN MIND & BODY ACTIONS AT HOME, WORK, SPORTS
HUMAN OBESITY: TREATMENT & THERAPY
HUMAN PREGNANCY COMPLICATIONS

HUMAN PSYCHOLOGY OF SINGLE PERSON
HUMAN RIGHTS
HUMAN RIGHTS & JURISPRUDENCE
HUMAN RIGHTS & SOCIAL JUSTICE

NEW REFERENCE BOOKS & RESEARCH INDEXES

GRADUATE EDUCATION AND ITS RESEARCH
IS A POTENTIAL CAULDRON
OF
CREATIVITY.

HUMAN RIGHTS TO DIE

HUMAN SEX BEHAVIOR
HUMAN STRESS & DISTRESS: PSY & MED THER
HUMAN STRESS & ESCAPE REACTIONS
HUNGER
HYDROXYBENZOIC ACIDS

HYPERTENSION
HYPNOSIS
HYPOGLYCEMIA
IATROGENIC DISEASES 1
IMMIGRATION & EMIGRATION
IMPOTENCE

INCEST: ACTS, MYTHS & FACTS

INDIANS OF NORTH AMERICA
INDUSTRY & HEALTH AFFAIRS

INFANT FOOD & NUTRITION OF NEWBORN
INFECTION & INFECTIONS
INFECTIONS BY HOOKWORMS
INFECTIOUS SKIN DISEASES
INFLAMMATION
INFORMATION SERVICES FOR THE WORLD
INFORMATION SYSTEMS
INJURIES & WOUNDS 1
INJURIES OF THE SPINAL CORD

INSOMNIA
INSTITUTIONALIZATION
INSURANCE & ECONOMIC VALUES OF LIFE
INSURANCE LIABILITY

INSURANCE LIABILITY & LEGAL IMPLICATIONS
INTELLIGENCE
INTELLIGENCE TESTS
INTERIOR DESIGN & FURNISHINGS
INTERNAL MEDICINE
INTL BIBLIOGRAPHY: CRIME PUBLICATIONS
INTL COOPERATION IN MED & SCIENCE

NEW REFERENCE BOOKS & RESEARCH INDEXES

RESEARCH KEEPS WORMS AND MANY TYPES OF PARASITES OUT OF OUR BODIES.

INTERNSHIP & RESIDENCY
INTERPERSONAL RELATIONS

INTRA-UTERINE DEVICES
INVERTEBRATES

JEWS & ETHNIC FACTORS
JEWS, JUDAISM & THE HOLOCAUST

JURISPRUDENCE
JURISPRUDENCE & ASBESTOS
JURISPRUDENCE & CHILD ABUSE PREVENTION
JURISPRUDENCE & CLINICAL COMPETENCE
JURISPRUDENCE & CONFIDENTIALITY

JURISPRUDENCE & CONSUMER PRODUCT SAFETY
JURISPRUDENCE & CRIME
JURISPRUDENCE & CRIME ANALYSIS

JURISPRUDENCE & DIAGNOSTIC ERRORS

JURISPRUDENCE & DOCTOR-CAUSED DISEASES
JURISPRUDENCE & DRUG-NARCOTIC CONTROL
JURISPRUDENCE & EXPERT TESTIMONY
JURISPRUDENCE & FORENSIC TECHNOLOGY
JURISPRUDENCE & FORENSICS
JURISPRUDENCE & GOVERNMENT FINANCING
JURISPRUDENCE & HIV INFECTED CARE PERSONNEL

JURISPRUDENCE & WRONGFUL BIRTHS, NEGLIGENCE
JURISPRUDENCE & IATROGENIC (DOCTOR) PROBLEMS
JURISPRUDENCE & INFORMED CONSENT
JURISPRUDENCE & INSURANCE LIABILITY
JURISPRUDENCE & LIFE SUPPORT CARE
JURISPRUDENCE & MED EQUIPMENT SAFETY & FAIL
JURISPRUDENCE & MEDICAL MALPRACTICE

JURISPRUDENCE & MEDICAL MISTAKES
JURISPRUDENCE & MEDICATION ERRORS
JURISPRUDENCE & OCCUPATIONAL HEALTH
JURISPRUDENCE & ORGAN PROCUREMENTS

NEW REFERENCE BOOKS & RESEARCH INDEXES

MANY OF US TODAY WOULD NOT BE ALIVE
        BUT
            FOR RESEARCH MADE ON
                        ANTIBIOTICS.

JURISPRUDENCE & PATIENT ADVOCACY
JURISPRUDENCE & RIGHTS TO TREATMENT
JURISPRUDENCE & SUBSTANCE ABUSE DETECTION
JURISPRUDENCE & HEALTH SCIENCES
JURISPRUDENCE & TRUTH DISCLOSURES
JURISPRUDENCE IN HEALTH AFFAIRS

JURISPRUDENCE IN HEALTH BIOLOGY
JURISPRUDENCE, AIDS, HIV & TRUTH DISCLOSURES
JURISPRUDENCE, MED RECORDS & SYSTEMS

JURISPRUDENCE, PRODUCT SAFETY & LIABILITY
JURISPRUDENCE, RIGHTS TO TREATMENTS IN PRISON
JUVENILE DELINQUENCY

JURISPRUDENCE & PATIENT ADVOCACY
JURISPRUDENCE & RIGHTS TO TREATMENT
JURISPRUDENCE & SUBSTANCE ABUSE DETECTION
JURISPRUDENCE & HEALTH SCIENCES
JURISPRUDENCE & TRUTH DISCLOSURES
JURISPRUDENCE IN HEALTH AFFAIRS

KIDNEY TRANSPLANTATION
KNEE INJURIES

LABOR IN PREGNANCY
LABORATORY DIAGNOSIS

LANGUAGE & ITS FORMS AT WORK & PLAY USA

LASERS IN MED, SCIENCE & BIOLOGY
LEARNING DISORDERS
LEG INJURIES

LEGAL & MED LIABILITY IN HEALTH SCIENCES
LEGAL LIABILITY & MALPRACTICE IN HEALTH SCIENCE
LEGISLATION IN HEALTH SCIENCES
LEPROSY

LESBIANISM

LIBRARIES

NEW RESEARCH BOOKS & RESEARCH INDEXES

OH !! DEVELOPMENT OF A NATION
            CAN BE MEASURED
            BY THE AMOUNT OF
            RESEARCH
                        THEY PRODUCE.

LIBRARIES IN HEALTH SERVICE
LICE & PEDICULOSIS

LIFE CHANGE EVENTS & HEALTH
LIPIDS
LITHIUM IN BIOLOGY & MEDICINE
LIVER DISEASES

LOVE & LIBIDO
LUMBAR VERTEBRAE & INJURIES
LUNG DISEASES

MAGIC, SUPERSTITIONS & FOLKLORE
MALARIA
MALOCCLUSION

MALPRACTICE I
MALPRACTICE II
MALPRACTICE IN HEALTH OCCUPATIONS

MAMMOGRAPHY IN HEALTH & MEDICINE
MAMMOGRAPHY OF THE BREAST
MANAGEMENT OF PERSONNEL IN HEALTH SCIENCE
MARINE BIOLOGY
MARRIAGE & MARITAL THERAPY
MARRIAGE THERAPY
MARRIAGE ANALYSIS, TREATMENT & RESULTS

MASSAGE
MATERIAL TESTING & BIOCOMPATIBILITY

MEAT & HEALTH

MEDICAL & HEALTH BUSINESS & COMPETITION
MEDICAL & HEALTH COSTS OF CARE, ILLNESS, ET
MEDICAL & HEALTH PRACTICES: DEFENSIVE MED
MEDICAL & LEGAL LIABILITY IN HEALTH SCIENCE
MEDICAL & PSYCHOLOGICAL STRESS
MED-PSY OF PERSUASIVE COMMUNICATION

MED REPORTS: EFFICIENCY & PERFORMANCE
MEDICAL (ABBE) TRIBULATIONS, SABOTAGE, MURDER

NEW REFERENCE BOOKS & RESEARCH INDEXES

PEOPLE DIE EARLIER IN NATIONS
                    THAT PRODUCE
                              LESS
RESEARCH
                    THAN
                              OTHER NATIONS.

ATTEMPT OF AUTHORS, LOSS OF SHIPMENTS,
SURVEILLANCE & POISONINGS
MEDICAL ANALYSIS & REVIEWS OF HIV
MEDICAL ART OF RELAXATION IN SICKNESS & H

MEDICAL ASPECTS; FOOD HANDLING
MEDICAL ASSISTANCE: TITLE 19

MEDICAL CARE OF POOR & INDIGENT
MEDICAL CATHETERS & CATHERIZATIONS: HARM, ERRORS,
PUNCTURES, MIGRATIONS DISPLACEMENTS &
COMPLICATIONS

MEDICAL CAUSES OF DEATHS IN HOSPITALS

MEDICAL CONSULTATIONS; PRACTICE, IMPORTANCE

MEDICAL DANGERS IN OUR DRINKING WATER
MEDICAL: DECISIONS: AS 'DO NOT RESUSCITATE'
MEDICAL DEVICES
MEDICAL DEVICES & EQUIP: FAILURE, CONTAMINATION
MEDICAL ECONOMICS
MEDICAL EDUCATION
MEDICAL EFFECTS OF FREE RADICALS
MEDICAL ELECTRONICS & INSTRUMENTATION

MEDICAL EMERGENCIES
MEDICAL ETHICS
MEDICAL GRADUATES OF FOREIGN NATIONS
MEDICAL HEALTH OF THE WORLD

MEDICAL HISTORY
MEDICAL HISTORY OF CURRENT, OLD WARS
MEDICAL IMITATIONS OF ILLNESS, PRETENSE
MEDICAL INDEX OF SEVERITY OF SICKNESS
MEDICAL JURIS & CRIMINAL LAW

MEDICAL JURIS & CRIMINAL LAW II
MEDICAL LIBRARIES; ROLES, CHALLENGES
MEDICAL MANUSCRIPTS, ANCIENT & MODERN
MEDICAL MASS SCREENING FOR H & DISEASE
MEDICAL MEASUREMENTS OF PAIN

NEW REFERENCE BOOKS & RESEARCH INDEXES

THE BEST STUDENTS AND CREATIVE MINDS
COME
FROM
TEACHING TYPES OF SCIENTISTS.

MEDICAL PERIODICALS: FUNCTIONS, STANDARDS

MEDICAL PHYSICIAN IMPAIRMENTS
MEDICAL POLITICS
MEDICAL PRACTICE, DEFENSE MED, LEGAL ISSUES

MEDICAL PRESCRIPTIONS; ABUSE, EVAL, HABITS
MED PSEC OF ALCOHOL DRINKING ADDICTION

MED PSEC OF CHARACTER & PERSONALITIES
MED PSEC OF HOMOSEXUALITY, MALE, FEMALE
MED PSEC OF PHYSICIANS
MED PSEC OF REGRESSION & FACE PERSONALITY
MED PSYCHOLOGY OF SPOUSE ABUSE
MED PSYCHOLOGY OF ID, EGO & SUPEREGO
MEDICAL PSYCHOSOMATIC

MED REACTION, TREATMENT " OVERDOSE SUBSTANCES
MEDICAL REFERRALS FOR PACT & BUSINESS
MED RESEARCH & JUNGLE OF SCIENCE: NEW SYSTEM
MED RESEARCH IN HEALTH SCIENCES

MEDICAL RESEARCH: NEW CATEGORY: OXIDATIVE STRESS
MEDICAL RESEARCH: NEW CATEGORY: OXIDANTS
MED RESEARCH OF COMBAT DISORDERS, DAG, PSEC
MED RESEARCH OF CURRENT, PAST WARS
MED RESEARCH ON RADON & CANCER

MED RESEARCH ON STUDENTS

MED RESEARCH SUPPORT: WHAT'S GOING ON IN U.S.A.
MEDICAL SCHOOLS: ACTIVITIES, TRENDS, PROGRESS
MED SCIENCE APPLIED TO CRIME MYSTERY

MED SCIENTISTS R ON WAR & WARS: HISTORIC OPERATED

MED STUDIES OF HALLUCINOGENS
MED STUDIES OF POLYGRAPHS & OTHER LIE DETECTORS

MED STUDIES OF SALIVA
MED SUB ANAL: GENERAL COUNSELING
MED SUB RES: IATROGENESIS & IATROGENIC DISEASES

NEW REFERENCE BOOKS & RESEARCH INDEXES

COLLEGES HAVE BETTER RATINGS
WHEN THEY
HAVE PRODUCTIVE
RESEARCH SCIENTISTS.

MED SUBJ RES: MED MALPRACTICE EXCLUD IATROLOGY

MED SUBJ RES CONCERNING COCAINE
MED SUBJ DIR & BIBL FOR PSYCHOSOMATIC MEDICINE

MEDICAL SYSTEMS ANALYSIS & MANAGEMENT
MEDICAL TECHNOLOGY
MED TREATMENT OF SELF & HYPOCHONDRIA

MED USES OF ANTIOXIDANTS FOR CANCER PREVENTION

MEDICAL WIT AND HUMOR
MEDICAL FACTORS IN HUMAN PERSONALITY DISORDERS
MEDICINE, PSEC & SCI IN AUTOMOBILE DRIVING

MENOPAUSE
MENSTRUATION DISORDERS

MENTAL & INTELLIGENCE TESTS
MENTAL DISORDERS
MENTAL FATIGUE -ANALYSIS, TESTS, ETC
MENTAL HEALTH
MENTAL HEALTH CARE IN PRISONS
MENTAL HEALTH SERVICES
MENTAL PROCESSES

MENTAL RETARDATION
METABOLISM WITH INBORN ERRORS

METALLURGY IN MED & INDUSTRY

METALS IN HEALTH, FOOD & POLLUTION

METALS-PHYSIOLOGY & METABOLISM

METEOROLOGY & WEATHER FACTORS
METHODS & INSTRUMENTATION FOR MED AUTOMAT
METHODS IN BEHAVIOR THERAPY

METHODS IN HYPNOSIS
MICROWAVES & RADIATION
MIGRAINE

NEW REFERENCE BOOKS & RESEARCH INDEXES

WITHOUT NEW RESEARCH WE WOULD LOSE DEVELOPMENTS OF THE LAST 500 YEARS.

MILITARY MEDICINE
MILK & MILK RESEARCH
MINERALS IN HEALTH, SCI & RESEARCH
MINN MULTI-PHASE PERSONALITY INVENTORY (MMPI)

MINOXIDIL (ROGAINE)
MMPI
MOLECULAR BIOLOGY IN HEALTH SCI

MORALE IN HEALTH, LIFE & WORK
MORALS & ISSUES

MULTIPLE SCLEROSIS
MUSCLE CONTRACTION
MUSCLES & DRUG EFFECTS
MUSCLES & PHYSIOLOGY

MUSIC, MUSICIANS & HEALTH INFLUENCES

MUTAGENS & MUTAGENICITY TESTS
MYCOSES
MYOCARDIAL INFARCTION WITH DIAGNOS
NEOPLASMS - PREVENTION & CONTROL
NEUROLOGY
NEURONS
NEUROTIC DISORDERS
NICOTINE

NOISE & ADVERSE EFFECTS ON HEALTH
NUCLEAR WARFARE
NURSE PRACTITIONERS
NUTRITION & MEDICINE
NUTRITION DISORDERS

NUTRITIONAL CONDITIONS: GOOD, BAD, DISEASED

OBESITY
OCCUPATIONAL DISEASES
OCCUPATIONAL MEDICINE

ONCOGENES
OPTOMETRY

NEW REFERENCE BOOKS & RESEARCH INDEXES

RESEARCH SCIENTISTS SEEK
THE HOLY GRAIL
OF PERFECTION
FOR ALL MANKIND.

ORAL HEALTH & HYGIENE
ORGAN DONATIONS & PROCUREMENTS
ORTHOPEDICS
ORTHOPSYCHIATRY
OSTEOPATHY
OSTEOPOROSIS
OSTEOPOROSIS -CONDITIONS & THERAPY

PACEMAKERS
PARAPSYCHOLOGY & CLAIRVOYANCE
PARKINSONISM & TARDIV DYSKINESIA
PATENTS & HEALTH SCIENCE

PATHOLOGY
PATIENTS
PEDIGREE STUDIES

PEDOPHILIA & SEX BEHAVIORS

PEPTIDES
PERCHLORETHYLENE (DRYCLEANER, ET)
PERIODONTAL DISEASES
PERIPHERAL NERVE INJURIES
PERSONALITY DISORDERS

PERSONALITY TESTS & INVENTORY
PERSONNEL MANAGEMENT

PESTICIDES
PESTICIDES & CANCER
PETROLEUM & MEDICINE

PETS & DOMESTIC ANIMALS
PHENOLS & MEDICINE
PHENYTOIN (DILANTIN)
PHILATELY & HEALTH SCIENCE
PHILOSOPHY IN MED, SCI & HEALTH

PHOBIAS & DISORDERS
PHOTOGRAPHY IN LIFE SCIENCE
PHYSICAL EDUCATION & TRAINING
PHYSICAL ENDURANCE

NEW REFERENCE BOOKS & RESEARCH INDEXES

WHEN YOU HELP PROMOTE RESEARCH –

YOU HELP PROTECT
YOUR FUTURE HEALTH.

PHYSICAL FITNESS
PHYSICAL FITNESS & SPORTS MED
PHYSICAL THERAPY & HEALTH

PHYSICIAN--PATIENT RELATIONS
PLASTICS IN MEDICINE, SCIENCE, LAW
PODIATRY
POISONING & MED

POLICE -HEALTH, RISKS, WORK, ET

POLITICAL SYSTEMS -PROG, REACT
POLITICS & BIOMEDICINE
POLYMERASE CHAIN REAC
POPULATION: CONTROL, SURVEILLANCE
POVERTY & CULTURAL DEPRIVATION
PREGNANCY: CARE & PHYSIOLOGY
PREJUDICE

PREMENSTRUAL SYNDROME
PREVENTIVE MEDICINE

PRISONERS
PRISONS
PROSTATE & MALE HEALTH
PROSTATE RESEARCH
PROTECTIVE DEViCES FOR SPORT & WORK

PROVERBS TWISTED WITH WIT & HUMOR
PROZAC (FLUOXETINE) SIDE EFFECTS
PSYCHIATRIC MODELS IN MED
PSYCHIATRIC NURSING

PSYCHIATRIC STATUS RATING SCALES
PSYCHIATRY & MEDICINE
PSYCHO-PHYSIOLOGIC DISORDERS
PSYCHO-PHYSIOLOGIC DISORDERS II
PSYCHO-PHYSIOLOGY & BIOFEEDBACK
PSYCHO-PHYSIOLOGY OF FATIGUE

PSYCHOLOGICAL ADAPTATION IN LIFE & WORK
PSYCHOLOGICAL DEPRIVATION

NEW REFERENCE BOOKS & RESEARCH INDEXES

*READING RESEARCH REVIEWS
                              OF A SUBJECT
            GIVES YOU
                        DECADES
        OF
          PROGRESS AND ADVANCEMENTS.

PSYCHOL IMPROVEMENTS WITH FOREIGN WORDS

PSYCHOLOGICAL TESTS

PSYCHOLOGICAL TESTS & TESTING
PSYCHOLOGY & A.I.D.S.

PSYCHOLOGY AND HEALTH
PSYCHOLOGY & ITS PRACTICE
PSYCHOLOGY & RESEARCH OF SELF CONCEPTS
PSYCHOLOGY & MED OF APPETITE DISORDERS

PSYCHOLOGY OF ALCOHOLISM

PSYCHOLOGY OF ANXIETY, WORRY, ETC
PSYCHOLOGY OF ATTACHMENT & BONDING

PSYCHOLOGY OF ATTEMPTED SUICIDE
PSYCHOL OF CORONARY & CARDIO-VAS DIS
PSYCHOLOGY OF HYPERTENSION
PSYCHOLOGY OF INDIANS OF N AMERICA
PSYCHOLOGY OF MENTAL DISORDERS

PSYCHOLOGY OF PAIN
PSYCHOLOGY OF PERCEPTIONS

PSYCHOLOGY OF SELF-AFFIRM & ASSERTIVENESS
PSYCHOLOGY OF STRESS & DISTRESS
PSYCHOLOGY OF TEMPERAMENT

PSYCHOLOGY OF FAMILY IN HEALTH, STRESS & DISEASE

PSYCHOLOGY OF WOMEN
PSYCHOLOGY, PARA-PSYCHOLOGY & CLAIRVOYANCE
PSYCHOMOTOR PERFORMANCES
PSYCHOTHERAPY

PUBLIC & SOCIAL POLICY
PUBLIC HEALTH
PUBLIC HEALTH: ADVANCES, PROBLEMS, RISKS, ET
PUBLIC HOUSING
PUBLIC OPINIONS YOU SHOULD KNOW ABOUT

NEW REFERENCE BOOKS & RESEARCH INDEXES

CREATIVITY REQUIRES THE CONSTANT FEEDING
OF
NEW KNOWLEDGE:
MOSTLY,
FROM RESEARCH

PUBLISHING IN THE LIFE SCIENCES: INDEX
PUBLISHING STANDARDS IN LIFE SCIENCE

PUBLISHING & SELLING YOUR OWN BOOK

PUNISHMENT: FORMS, FUNCTION, TRIALS, ET
QUALITY OF HEALTH CARE
QUESTIONNAIRES
QUESTIONNAIRES IN BIO-MED
RADIO & RADIO WAVES
RADIOTHERAPY
RADON

RAPE --HOW TO FIGHT, PREVENT, USE PROTECTIVE
        PSYCHOLOGY OR LATER IDENTIFY RAPIST

RAPE
RAPE & VIOLENCE
RAPE VICTIMS, OFFENDERS, TREATMENT, JURIS
RECENT ADVANCES IN COMPUTER SCIENCE

RED CROSS: GOALS & ROLES
REDUCING DIET
REFLEX & REFLEXES
REFUSE & GARBAGE DISPOSAL

REHABILITATION
RELAXATION TECHNIQUES

RELIGION & MEDICINE
RELIGION & PASTORAL CARE
RELIGION & PSYCHOLOGY
RELIGION & THE HIV-AIDS COMMUNITY
RELIGION WITH MED, PSY & PHILOSOPHY ASPEC
RELIGIOUS BELIEFS
REPRODUCTION

RESEARCH ON HEALTH
RESPIRATORY INSUFFICIENCY & THER
RESPIRATORY TRACT INFECTIONS

RESTAURANTS; CONDITIONS, SYNDROMES

NEW REFERENCE BOOKS & RESEARCH INDEXES

PEOPLE WITHOUT RESEARCH KNOWLEDGE
ARE SELDOM
THE
BEST TEACHERS.

RESUSCITATION

RUNNING
SARCOMAS
SCHIZOPHRENIA
SCHIZOPHRENIC PSYCHOLOGY

SCHOOLS--PROGRESS, ACTIVITIES & TRENDS

SCIENCE & MED OF AUTOPSY
SCIENCE & MED OF BACKACHE
SCIENCE & MED OF SPORTS
SCI, MED & PSYCHOLOGY OF AUTOMOBILES
SCI, MED & PSYCHOLOGY OF PERSONALITY
SCLEROSIS
SCOLIOSIS

SEASONS AND ITS WEATHER, VAR & MOOD PSYCHOL

SEAT BELTS
SECURITY MEASURES
SEEDS
SELENIUM
SELF HELP GROUPS
SEMICONDUCTORS
SEPTICEMIA

SEX & BISEXUALITY
SEX & ORGASM RESEARCH
SEX & PEYRONIE'S DISEASE (PENILE)
SEX & PROSTITUTION
SEX & PSYCHOLOGY OF SEX OFFENSES
SEX & PSYCHOSEXUAL DEVELOPMENT

SEX & SEXUAL HARASSMENT

SEX & THE BIOLOGY OF COITUS
SEX & TRANSSEXUALISM
SEX BEHAVIOR
SEX BEHAVIOR, HIV & AIDS
SEX COUNSELING
SEX DISORDERS
SEX EDUCATION

NEW REFERENCE BOOKS & RESEARCH INDEXES

CREATIVITY REQUIRES
THE CONSTANT FEEDING
OF GOOD STUDENTS
WITH NEW KNOWLEDGE:
ESPECIALLY SO
FROM RESEARCH

SEX OFFENSES
SEX RESEARCH & MED I
SEXUAL ABUSE OF CHILDREN

SEXUAL DEVIATIONS & PARAPHILIAS
SEXUALLY TRANSMITTED DISEASES
SHOCK
SKIN INJURIES
SKULL FRACTURES

SLEEP RESEARCH & POLYSOMNOGRAPHY

SMOKING

SOAPS & SURF ACTIVE AGENTS
SOCIAL BEHAVIOR
SOCIAL BEHAVIOR & MED
SOCIAL DISCRIMINATION & PREJUDICE
SOCIAL INTER-PERSONAL INTERACTIONS
SOCIAL PERCEPTIONS, IMPRESSIONS, MENTAL ACTIONS
SOCIAL PSYCHOLOGY
SOCIAL SECURITY

SOCIAL VALUES
SOCIAL WORK & HEALTH SCIENCES

SODIUM GLUTAMATE (M.S.G.)
SODIUM HYPOCHLORITE: USES, IMPORTANCE

SOLVENTS, NEW, USED, HAZARDOUS
SOVIET MILITARY MEDICINE

SPACE FLIGHT
SPACE FLIGHT & AEROSPACE MEDICIN

SPEECH

SPORTS: RESEARCH & GUIDEBOOK
SPORTS: GUIDEBOOK FOR REF & RES
SPORTS: INDEX OF MODERN DEVELOPMENTS
SPORTS & ANABOLIC STEROIDS

NEW REFERENCE BOOKS & RESEARCH INDEXES

WHERE THERE IS LESS RESEARCH
                                    THERE IS
        MORE SICKNESS,
                    GREATER SPREAD OF DISEASE
        AND CONSTANT
                    POVERTY
                        AND
                            AN UNHAPPY POPULATION

SPORTS & ATHLETIC INJURIES
SPORTS & BLOOD PRESSURE
SPORTS & COMPETITIVE BEHAVIOR
SPORTS & HEART RATE
SPORTS & NEW EXERCISE RESEARCH

SPORTS & PSYCHO-PHYSIOLOGY

SPORTS & PSYCHOLOGICAL INFLUENCES

SPORTS - MENTAL HEALTH, PSYCHIC STRESS, EMOTIONAL
        REACTIONS
SPORTS -PERFORMANCE & CIRCADIAN RHYTHMS
SPORTS PERFORMANCE: ANALYSIS, SKILLS, TRNG, ET

SPORTS REPORT: BASEBALL
SPORTS REPORT: FOOTBALL
SPORTS REPORT: SOCCER
SPORTS REPORT: SWIMMING

SPORTS REPORT: TENNIS
SPORTS REPORT: TENNIS ELBOW
SPORTS REPORT: TRACK & FIELD
SPORTS WITH RACQUETS (BADMINTON, RACQUETBALL &
        SQUASH)

SPORTS, DRUGS & DOPING

SPORTS, EXERCISE & ENERGY METABOLISM IN MEN AND
        WOMEN
SPORTS; PREVENTION, CONTROL OF ATHLETE INJURIES
STAMPS & PHILATELY HONORS IN SCI & MED

STERILIZATION & DISINFECTION
STRESS
STRESS DISORDERS IN POST-TRAUMA
SUDDEN DEATH

SUICIDE
SUICIDE & ITS PSYCHOLOGICAL INFLUENCES
SUICIDE PREVENTION & CONTROL
SUICIDE WITH ASSISTANCE

NEW REFERENCE BOOKS & RESEARCH INDEXES

RESEARCH IS SO IMPORTANT IT SHOULD BE MADE
A UNIVERSAL LAW
FOR ALL
UNIVERSITIES,
STUDENTS, TEACHERS AND FACULTIES.

SURGERY
SWIMMING

TEACHING: ACTIONS, METHODS, ETC
TECHNOLOGY ASSESSMENTS

TELECOMMUNICATIONS

TELEVISION IN MED & SCIENCE

TERATOGENS
THERAPEUTIC MATERIALS
THERAPEUTIC USES ANTI-OXIDANTS FOR HEALTH
      IMPROVEMTS
THERAPY MADE EASY WITH COMPUTER ASSIST

THERAPY OF ALCOHOLISM
THERAPY OF ANXIETY & CHRONIC WORRY

THERAPY OF MENTAL DISORDERS
THROMBOSIS
TISSUE DONATIONS & POST-M GIFTS
TOBACCO

TOBACCO SMOKE IN ACTIVE & PASSIVE POLLUTION

TOURETTE'S SYNDROME

TOXIC SUBSTANCES IN HEALTH BIOL
TOXICOLOGY I

TRACE ELEMENTS IN HEALTH BIOL

TRAFFIC ACCIDENTS
TRANQUILIZING AGENTS, ADVERSE EFFECTS
TRAVEL -BENEFITS & DANGERS, RISKS, WARNINGS, ET
TRETINOIN: ACTIONS, HARMFUL REACTIONS

TYPE A PERSONALITY   U.S.
CENTERS FOR DISEASE CONTROL

NEW REFERENCE BOOKS AND RESEARCH INDEXES

ALL NATIONS HAVE MANY SINS:
ONE SUCH:
POOR TEACHING EVERYWHERE
AND LACK
OF
THOROUGH TRAINING OF STUDENTS.

U.S. FOOD & DRUG ADMINISTRATION
ULTRASONIC DIAGNOSIS
ULTRAVIOLET RAYS & ADVERSE EFFECT
UNIVERSITY MALPRACTICE: ESSAYS
URINALYSIS: METHODS, DIAGN, STD & ABUSE INJURY
URINE & POLYMEDICINE: GUIDEBOOK
URINE STUDIES IN LABS & PRACTICE

VAGINITIS
VASECTOMY

VEGETABLES & HEALTH SCIENCE
VEGETARIANISM
VENEREAL DISEASES
VETERANS: CASES, OUTCOMES, ET

VETERINARIANS' NEW RESEARCH BIBLE
VETERINARY MEDICINE
VETERINARIANS' NEW RESEARCH BIBLE

VIDEOS: USES, METHODS
VIOLENCE: PSYCHOLOGY, MED & LEGAL ASPECTS
VIRUS DISEASES
VIRUSES

VITAMIN DEFICIENCIES
VITAMIN P COMPLEX (BIOFLAVANOIDS)
VITAMINS
VITAMINS & MEDICINE

VOLUNTEER HEALTH AGENCIES & WORKERS

WAR: MEDICAL, PSYCHOL, SCIENTIFIC ANALYSIS
WAR WITH MILITARY & CIVIL ASPECTS
WEATHER, HEALTH & BIOMEDICAL ASPECTS
WECHSLER SCALES

WHIPLASH INJURIES

NEW REFERENCE BOOKS AND RESEARCH INDEXES

WITHOUT STRICT DISCIPLINE IN SCHOOLS,
                    WARS,
               DISEASE, POVERTY
                    AND
               MASS IGNORANCE
                         WILL CONTINUE FOREVER....

WOMEN & PELVIC INFLAMMATORY DIS
WOMEN & SPOUSE ABUSE
WOMEN & TAMPONS

WOMEN & THEIR LIFE-STYLES
WOMEN & VAGINA RESEARCH

WOMEN & WOMEN'S RIGHTS
WOMEN'S BIBLIOGRAPHY OF CONCERNS, ETC
WOMEN'S HEALTH SERVICES

WORK, INJURIES & COMPENSATION
WORK, JOBS, DISTRESS, DANGERS & DISEASE

WORKMAN'S COMPENSATION

WORLD HEALTH & THE W.H.O.
WOUND HEALING
YIN DEFICIENCY & YIN-YANG
YOGA
ZIDOVUDINE IN THERAPEUTIC USE

ZOONOSES & MEDICINE
ZYMONAS